Understanding
Heart Failure

Professor John Cleland

Published by Family Doctor Publications Limited
in association with the British Medical Association

IMPORTANT
This book is intended not as a substitute for personal
medical advice but as a supplement to that advice for
the patient who wishes to understand more about his
or her condition.

Before taking any form of treatment
YOU SHOULD ALWAYS CONSULT YOUR MEDICAL
PRACTITIONER.

In particular (without limit) you should note that
advances in medical science occur rapidly and some
information about drugs and treatment contained in this
booklet may very soon be out of date.

© Family Doctor Publications 2000–2008
Updated 2003, 2005, 2008

Family Doctor Publications, PO Box 4664, Poole, Dorset BH15 1NN

ISBN-13: 978 1 903474 15 0
ISBN-10: 1 903474 15 9

Contents

About the author

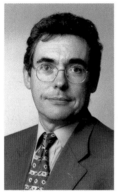 **Professor John Cleland** is head of the Department of Academic Cardiology, University of Hull – an international centre for research into and management of heart failure. He is Editor-in-Chief of the *European Journal of Heart Failure* and leader of several national and international research programmes bringing new understanding and treatment of patients with this condition.

What is heart failure?

Case history: Eric

Eric was 67 when he was taken to hospital with severe pains in the middle of his chest. Tests showed that he'd had a heart attack. He recovered over the next 10 days without any further major problems, but felt exhausted most of the time.

In the following months he noticed that he was getting more and more breathless, even walking at a gentle pace. Three months after his heart attack, he found that he could no longer walk even to the newsagents without stopping to catch his breath.

Eric went to see his GP, who examined him. His GP suspected that he might have heart failure, took a blood test (to check for anaemia or a kidney problem), organised a special test at the local hospital (an echocardiogram) and gave him some water tablets.

Over the next few days Eric passed a lot more urine, lost two and a half kilograms (four to five pounds) in weight and his breathlessness greatly improved. The hospital test confirmed that he had developed heart failure as a result of the heart attack and that further treatment could help to keep the problem under control.

Heart failure: what is it?

The heart is a sophisticated muscular pump that is designed to push blood around the arteries of the body at a high enough pressure for the needs of organs such as the brain and kidney, while keeping the pressure in the veins (the vessels that take the blood back to the heart) low.

Heart failure means that the heart is not keeping up with all these varied demands, leading either to:

- a rise in the blood pressure in the veins or
- a fall in the amount of blood pumped by the heart.

Increased pressure in the veins of the lungs leads to breathlessness and in the veins of the legs to swelling of the ankles. The cause of these symptoms will be explained more fully later.

Reduced blood flow may be responsible for fatigue and cause the kidneys to retain salt and water, which then leads to more fluid gathering in the lungs and ankles. In order to cope, the heart requires medical help, usually in the form of pills which help to get rid of the extra salt and water and enable the heart to work more effectively.

On medical therapy (treatment with medicines), some people with heart failure will feel entirely well and many people will be able to lead relatively normal lives. However, not all patients respond to existing treatments. Medical research on heart failure has probably been more successful in improving patients' lives than for any other medical condition in the last decade. Research continues to produce about one major medical advance each year for patients with heart failure.

Heart failure can be the end-result of many different heart problems so it is important to find out why it has happened. The most common causes of heart failure are coronary artery disease, high blood pressure and a heart rhythm problem called atrial fibrillation. These problems are discussed in detail later.

There are many other rarer causes of heart failure, some needing different treatments, so it is important for your doctor to find out the cause in your particular case. In most cases, medication can help to improve the action of the heart and relieve the symptoms of heart failure.

Heart failure

- Means that the heart can no longer do its work properly without some medical help
- With medical help symptoms may be controlled and quality of life maintained for many years
- Over 100,000 people develop heart failure in the UK each year
- At any time, about 1 million people in the UK will have some form of heart failure

Symptoms of heart failure

The main symptoms are breathlessness, swollen ankles and tiredness, but there can be many other reasons for this combination of symptoms and attempts at self-diagnosis are often incorrect. Your doctor must make the diagnosis for you.

How severe the symptoms are depends on the amount of damage done to the heart. The main symptoms are listed briefly in the box, but we will look at symptoms in detail in the chapter starting on page 36. However, it is important to remember that no two people are likely to have exactly the same combination of symptoms and some will have more problems than others.

Who gets heart failure?

Heart failure is uncommon in people under the age of 50, but it affects progressively more people in older age groups. The principal cause of heart failure between the ages of 50 and 75 is coronary artery disease that has led to a heart attack. A heart attack means that one of the blood vessels taking oxygen to the heart muscle becomes blocked. As a result, part of the heart muscle dies, leaving a scar. So anything that makes a heart attack more likely also increases the risk of heart failure. This means that people who smoke, or who have high blood pressure, high blood cholesterol or diabetes are more likely to develop heart failure.

It is also possible for heart failure to occur without being preceded by a heart attack, especially in older people. This may also be the result of coronary artery disease or prolonged and/or severe high blood pressure or atrial fibrillation.

Narrowed or leaking heart valves may cause heart failure in people of any age but are also more common in older people.

Occasionally, drinking excessive amounts of alcohol can poison the heart muscle. Abstinence from alcohol may allow a partial or even a full recovery.

Rarer causes of heart failure may affect pregnant women and people with muscular dystrophy and, more

Symptom guide for heart failure

A person with heart failure may have one or more of the following symptoms, but other medical problems can cause similar symptoms:

- Shortness of breath which gets worse during exercise or with lying flat
- Needing to sleep sitting up or waking at night with severe breathlessness
- Coughing and wheezing, especially at night
- Swollen ankles and weight gain caused by retention of fluid
- Passing lots of urine at night (sometimes the body can get rid of fluid retained during the day when you lie down)
- Unexplained weight loss
- Tiredness

rarely still, children and unborn babies can get heart failure.

Case history: Ken

Ken, a widower aged 75, had been well until he started having problems getting about because of his shortness of breath. He found that he could no longer climb stairs or hurry for the bus without getting out of breath. He went to his GP, who told him that there was some fluid on his lungs and prescribed water tablets (diuretics) to clear it. Before long, Ken was feeling much more like his old self. An echocardiography test (see page 46) at the local hospital showed a narrowed heart (aortic) valve. Three months after valve replacement he is back to normal.

Case history: Lily

Lily, an 81-year-old woman, was brought by her daughter to see her GP because she was worried that her mother seemed to be getting very tired, with swollen ankles and breathlessness, and was becoming confused at night. She had enjoyed good health until recently apart from long-standing (15 years) high blood pressure, for which she had been given treatment, although she had often forgotten to take it.

The doctor suggested that heart failure resulting from the high blood pressure might be the cause of all her problems, including the confusion. He arranged for an echocardiogram at the local hospital which showed that the heart had indeed been damaged by the high blood pressure.

Treatment with water pills and a medicine called an angiotensin-converting enzyme (ACE) inhibitor rapidly improved her symptoms, including her confusion.

Case history: Irene

Irene had a heart attack two years ago and for the last few months she'd been having symptoms that gradually got worse. Her ankles were often very swollen and she was short of breath. Recently she'd started waking in the night unable to get her breath.

Her GP arranged for her to see the specialist at the hospital outpatient department. Tests confirmed heart failure. The patient responded well to a combination of medicines including a beta blocker, ACE inhibitor and water pill (diuretic).

KEY POINTS

■ Heart attacks, high blood pressure and atrial fibrillation are the most common reasons for people to develop heart failure

■ Highly effective treatments for these conditions exist that may prevent heart failure from developing or treat it effectively when it appears

How your heart works

The cardiovascular system

Together, the heart and all the blood vessels around the body form the cardiovascular system. Your heart is a pump made of muscle. It is made from a special type of muscle not found anywhere else in the body, so it doesn't get tired the way that ordinary muscles do. Its task is to keep your body supplied with the nutrients and oxygen that are dissolved in your blood.

The arteries carry the blood away from the heart and the veins bring it back; the direction of blood flow through the heart is controlled by valves which open to let blood through, then close tightly to prevent it going back the wrong way.

The average person has about five litres (eight pints) of blood, which circulate around the body in about one minute while you're at rest. When you exert yourself physically, your heart speeds up and pumps harder, and may pump as much as 20 or 30 litres in a minute. A failing heart is not capable of doing this, which is why vigorous exercise of any kind becomes difficult.

Cardiovascular system

Diagram showing the heart and circulation with veins (blue) draining the blood back to the heart where it is pumped to the lungs and back to the rest of the body through the arteries (red). Larger blood vessels branch into smaller and smaller ones and then to tiny networks of blood vessels known as capillaries, where oxygen and nutrients are passed from the blood into the surrounding cells.

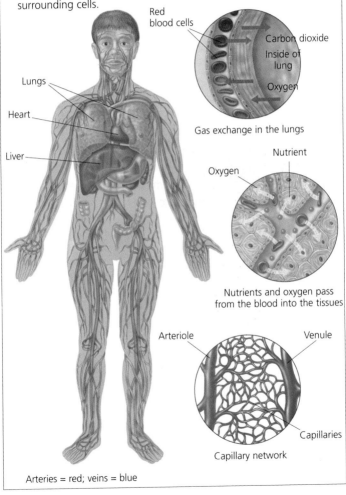

Red blood cells

Carbon dioxide

Inside of lung

Oxygen

Gas exchange in the lungs

Lungs

Heart

Liver

Nutrient

Oxygen

Nutrients and oxygen pass from the blood into the tissues

Arteriole

Venule

Capillaries

Capillary network

Arteries = red; veins = blue

The pumping cycle of the heart

The heart is a muscular organ, acting as a pump. The heart consists of four chambers which work together in a cycle as two pairs.

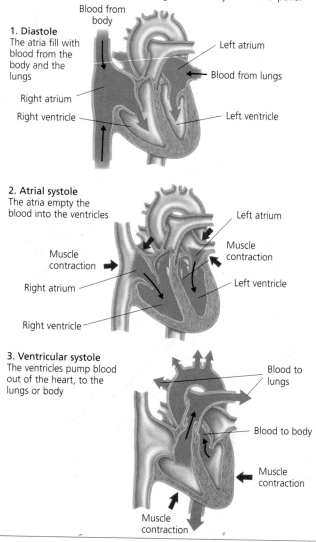

1. Diastole
The atria fill with blood from the body and the lungs

Blood from body

Left atrium

Blood from lungs

Right atrium

Right ventricle

Left ventricle

2. Atrial systole
The atria empty the blood into the ventricles

Left atrium

Muscle contraction

Muscle contraction

Right atrium

Left ventricle

Right ventricle

3. Ventricular systole
The ventricles pump blood out of the heart, to the lungs or body

Blood to lungs

Blood to body

Muscle contraction

Muscle contraction

The heart is divided into separate halves which beat together but pump blood to different parts of the body. The right side receives 'used' blood, low in oxygen, from the body and sends it off to the lungs to be replenished with oxygen. The left side receives the oxygenated blood from the lungs and pumps it around the body.

Each side of the heart has an upper and lower chamber. The upper ones, called the atria, are where blood is collected from the veins. They are designed to operate at low pressure. When valves leading to the lower chambers (the ventricles) open, the atria contract, emptying the blood into the ventricles. Those valves close and the exit valves into the arteries open. The ventricles then contract in their turn and the blood is pumped out into the arteries at much higher pressure than in the veins.

Arteries are the vessels that take blood from the ventricles to either the body (the systemic arteries) or the lungs (pulmonary arteries). They are thick walled in order to contain the relatively high pressure generated by the ventricles. The blood in the systemic arteries is usually bright red because it is oxygen rich and if an artery is punctured the blood will spurt out.

The veins take blood back from the body or lungs to the atria at low pressure. The veins are thin walled. The blood in the systemic veins is usually dark and, if a vein is damaged, blood oozes out. Both arteries and veins branch like trees from the heart and end up as tiny vessels in the tissues.

Microscopic vessels, called capillaries, connect the smallest arteries and veins. If you scratch yourself, the blood usually comes from capillaries and is bright red. The capillary walls are only one cell thick and they allow oxygen, fluid, nutrients and waste to be exchanged between the circulation and the tissues.

The heart and great vessels

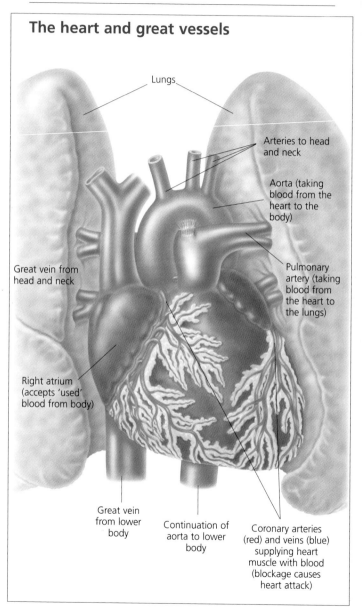

Lungs

Arteries to head and neck

Aorta (taking blood from the heart to the body)

Pulmonary artery (taking blood from the heart to the lungs)

Great vein from head and neck

Right atrium (accepts 'used' blood from body)

Great vein from lower body

Continuation of aorta to lower body

Coronary arteries (red) and veins (blue) supplying heart muscle with blood (blockage causes heart attack)

Internal anatomy of the heart

Arrows indicate direction of blood flow.

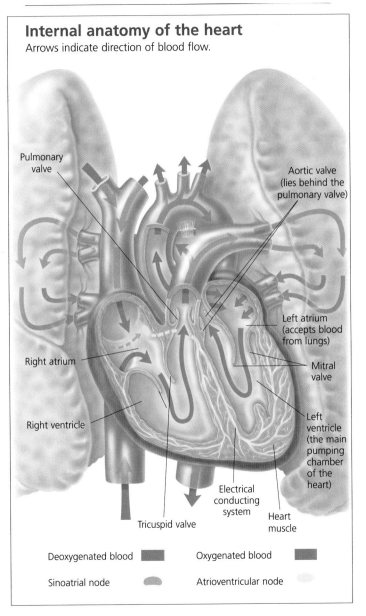

Pulmonary valve

Aortic valve (lies behind the pulmonary valve)

Left atrium (accepts blood from lungs)

Right atrium

Mitral valve

Right ventricle

Left ventricle (the main pumping chamber of the heart)

Electrical conducting system

Heart muscle

Tricuspid valve

Deoxygenated blood

Oxygenated blood

Sinoatrial node

Atrioventricular node

13

Capillaries

Microscopic vessels called capillaries connect the smallest arteries and veins. Their walls are very thin and allow oxygen and nutrients to pass into and nourish the tissue cells.

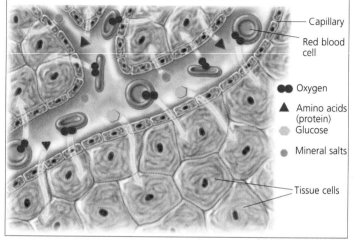

- Capillary
- Red blood cell
- ●● Oxygen
- ▲ Amino acids (protein)
- Glucose
- Mineral salts
- Tissue cells

The term 'blood pressure' usually refers to the pressure in the arteries. With each beat (pump) of the heart, pressure rises to a high point (systolic pressure), then falls to its lowest point between beats (diastolic pressure). Both are measured using a device called a sphygmomanometer and recorded as millimetres of mercury (or mmHg). Recently small electronic desktop devices that do not use mercury are being used for blood pressure measurement. Most people will have had this test done at some time.

Taking blood pressure involves putting an inflating cuff around your upper arm. As the cuff around your arm is inflated, it eventually tightens sufficiently to stop the blood flow in the lower arm for a few seconds. The air is then let out, gradually lowering the pressure in the cuff, while the doctor, nurse or the machine itself

Blood pressure

Blood pressure is the pressure within the arteries as the heart forces blood to circulate around your body.

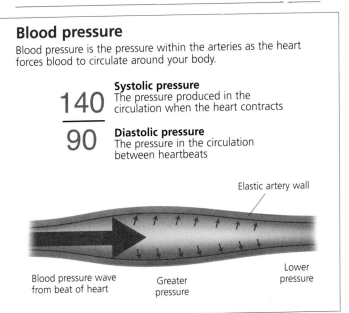

140 Systolic pressure
The pressure produced in the circulation when the heart contracts

90 Diastolic pressure
The pressure in the circulation between heartbeats

Elastic artery wall

Blood pressure wave from beat of heart

Greater pressure

Lower pressure

listens to the artery at the elbow for the sounds made by the blood as the flow returns to normal. The two pressures – systolic and diastolic – are usually expressed as, for example, 170/90 or 170 over 90. A healthy young person's blood pressure should be around 120/70; in older people, 140/90 is a borderline increase and 150/100 is definitely raised. In people with diabetes, the guidelines are to reduce blood pressure to 130/80

The contractions of both the upper and the lower chambers of the heart are controlled by a network of special electrical tissue throughout the heart. An area in the right atrium, called the sinus node, acts as a natural pacemaker, ensuring that the heart beats regularly and evenly. After a short delay, the electrical signal then passes down a 'wire' to the ventricles. The electrical signal fans out across the ventricles like the branches of a tree, causing them to contract in a coordinated fashion after the atria have finished contracting. This coordinated action is very important for the efficiency of the heart.

In order to do its job properly, your heart muscle must be able to pump, the valves should be neither leaking nor narrowed, and the pumping action must happen in a coordinated fashion. Failure of any one of these functions may lead to heart failure. Most patients with heart failure will have more than one of these problems.

When the heart starts to fail . . .

When the heart starts to fail, four important changes occur (see box). Highly effective treatments for this problem exist, which may prevent heart failure from developing or treat it effectively when it appears.

The fall in the output of the heart activates nerves and hormones (chemical messengers in the blood) that lead the kidneys to retain salt and water and alter blood vessel function. Curiously both the signals that cause blood vessels to constrict and also to relax are activated, although constriction usually predominates.

Key consequences of heart failure

1. A fall in the amount of blood pumped out by the heart (especially during exercise)
2. A rise in pressure in the atria and veins as blood is 'backed up' behind the failing heart
3. Salt and water retention by the kidneys
4. Constriction of arteries and veins

As a result the output of the heart is reduced and the muscles of the body may not receive enough oxygen and nutrients or may not be cleared of waste products, leading to tiredness.

As a result of a rise in pressure in the atria and veins and of salt and water retention, the pressure rises in the tiny blood vessels in the tissues (called capillaries). These start to leak fluid out into the tissues. Fluid can then collect in the lungs, causing breathlessness, or in the legs. When fluid leaks into the lungs it takes up space that should have been filled with air, reducing the amount of oxygen reaching the blood, and so the person becomes short of breath.

The reason that fluid gathers in the legs during the day is a result of the effect of gravity, which is why ankle swelling is worst in the evening (after a day of standing) and has often resolved in the morning (after a period of lying flat). The fluid from the legs gets re-distributed when you lie down and so the kidneys are able to deal with it more easily.

There are many different types of medications for treating heart failure and, as they work in different ways, they can often be combined. Some work by correcting or controlling the underlying problem, some control symptoms and some do both. We will look more closely at the symptoms of heart failure on page 36 and at how some of these medicines work on page 51.

KEY POINTS

■ Your heart is a pump made of muscle

■ The average person has about five litres of blood circulating round the body in one minute when at rest

■ A failing heart cannot pump harder which is why vigorous exercise is difficult

What causes heart failure?

The different causes of heart failure

There are many causes of heart failure and most patients will have more than one cause. Which cause is most likely or important depends on the age of the individual concerned. The following is a simple classification of the causes of heart failure (a more detailed one will follow), useful for people with or without medical training:

- Weak hearts: generally caused by coronary artery disease and heart attacks or more rarely dilated cardiomyopathy (the heart has become large and pumps weakly). Experts call this left ventricular systolic dysfunction

- Stiff hearts: generally in older people, especially women, and often caused by long-standing high blood pressure. Experts call this left ventricular diastolic dysfunction or heart failure with preserved systolic function

- Overloaded hearts: caused by problems such as a narrowed valve (often aortic) or very high blood pressure or anaemia (reduced number of blood cells), which requires the heart to pump more blood in order to deliver the same amount of oxygen to the tissues

- Leaking hearts: caused by leaking heart valves
- Confused hearts: confused either because they have a chaotic rhythm or because the contraction of the walls of the ventricles has lost coordination.

Coronary artery disease

Coronary artery disease may cause heart failure in several ways but the most common is by the development of a heart attack. Coronary disease is caused by the accumulation of cholesterol in the walls of the arteries supplying the heart muscle with blood. The cholesterol leads to atheroma, which means fatty deposits of cholesterol along with dead and dying cells; this leads to low-grade inflammation as the body tries but fails to clear up the mess.

Atheroma furs up the artery like lime-scale in a pipe, eventually blocking the free flow of blood. This can cause angina (heart pain) or, if very severe, it can cause the heart muscle to stop contracting.

If one of the lumps of atheroma cracks this can trigger bleeding into the artery wall and a blood clot then forms, leading to a heart attack, also known as a 'coronary' or a 'myocardial infarction'.

Risk factors for developing coronary disease include smoking, high blood pressure, diabetes and genetic factors (that is, a family history of heart attacks).

Heart attack

A heart attack is the most common cause of heart failure in people between the ages of 50 and 75 years.

Coronary artery disease and atheroma

Atheroma may block the coronary arteries and cause a heart attack.

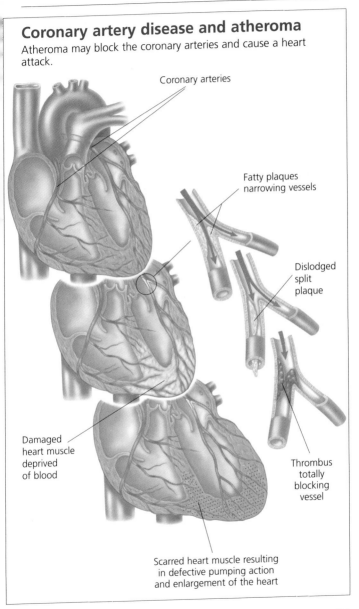

Coronary arteries

Fatty plaques narrowing vessels

Dislodged split plaque

Damaged heart muscle deprived of blood

Thrombus totally blocking vessel

Scarred heart muscle resulting in defective pumping action and enlargement of the heart

In a heart attack, one or more of the blood vessels taking oxygen to the heart muscle become blocked by a blood clot. This is why the so-called 'clot-busting' medicines are often used to treat heart attacks.

As a result of being starved of oxygen part of the heart muscle dies, which will then be replaced by a scar that cannot contract when the rest of the muscle does. The scar may gradually stretch, leading to enlargement of the heart, which then puts an extra strain on the undamaged heart muscle. This interferes with the efficient working of the heart and may lead to heart failure. Prompt hospital treatment with appropriate medicines (see page 52) can, if given in the first few hours after the attack, reduce the amount of damage done and improve the healing process.

The amount of heart muscle that is damaged in large part determines whether the person will develop heart failure. Occasionally, a heart attack can damage the muscle that supports the mitral valve (see diagram on page 13), causing the valve to leak. This can also lead to heart failure.

Roughly one person in every three who has a heart attack will show some evidence of heart failure. In some people, it may be mild and perhaps only temporary. Around one in five of those who do not have any problems initially will go on to develop heart failure in the next five or ten years, although treatment may prevent or at least delay it. Unfortunately, in some people damage to the heart muscle is so extensive that severe heart failure develops rapidly and may be difficult to control.

High blood pressure

Most people with high blood pressure have what is known as 'essential hypertension' – that is, their blood pressure is raised for no apparent reason. The triggering factors for essential hypertension are unclear, but obesity, high salt intake and high cholesterol may play a role. Less commonly, high blood pressure is caused by kidney disease or diseases of other glands.

Someone with high blood pressure will probably have no symptoms at all, which is why it is important to have regular checks. If your blood pressure is found to be raised, your doctor will probably repeat the test several times over the next few weeks and, if it stays high, you'll be put on long-term medication to bring it down. You must keep taking the tablets, even though you have no symptoms and can't feel any benefit; unless your blood pressure is kept under control, it could eventually damage your heart and it also increases the risk of a stroke.

The higher the pressure, the harder the heart has to work. Not only does raised blood pressure make an important contribution to the development of coronary disease, it may also cause heart failure in older people who have never actually had a heart attack and even occasionally in younger people if it is high enough.

With prolonged high blood pressure the heart muscle gets thicker and more bulky as it continues to try to pump blood around the body. This thickened muscle is stiffer and functions less well than normal heart muscle. High pressure also damages the walls of the arteries over time. They become stiffer, and this in turn raises the pressure in the system further, increasing the risk of a heart attack or stroke.

All this takes place gradually over many years, so the earlier high blood pressure is treated, the better the chances of delaying or even preventing the onset of heart failure or other complications of high blood pressure.

High blood pressure

High blood pressure can damage the heart muscle and walls of the arteries.

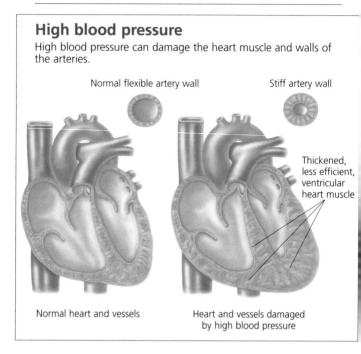

Normal flexible artery wall

Stiff artery wall

Thickened, less efficient, ventricular heart muscle

Normal heart and vessels

Heart and vessels damaged by high blood pressure

Even when heart failure has already developed, it's important to treat any coexisting high blood pressure, because this makes it easier for the heart to pump efficiently.

Atrial fibrillation

In this condition, the upper chambers of the heart (the atria) beat at a much faster rate than they should. The chaotic electrical impulses in the atria are transmitted to the lower chambers (the ventricles) which consequently also beat fast and irregularly. The heart chambers may not have time to fill properly or empty completely, reducing the amount of blood being pumped out and making the heart inefficient.

There are many possible reasons why atrial fibrillation may occur. It generally reflects either direct damage to the atria or increased back-pressure on the atria caused by damage to the ventricles, which is usually the result of coronary disease.

An overactive thyroid can cause atrial fibrillation. About a quarter of cases of heart failure are caused or complicated by atrial fibrillation. Atrial fibrillation increases the risk of blood clots forming in the heart and, if these clots break off, they may lodge in a blood

Atrial fibrillation

Atrial fibrillation increases the risk of blood clots forming in the heart which may cause a stroke. This diagram shows a clot forming in the left atrium, then causing a stroke.

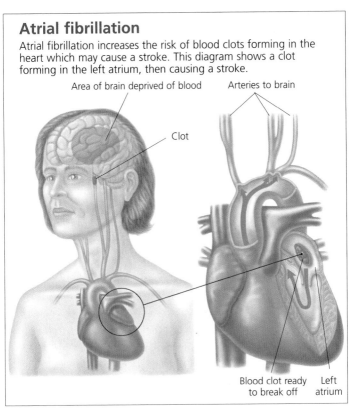

Area of brain deprived of blood

Arteries to brain

Clot

Blood clot ready to break off

Left atrium

vessel in part of the brain, starving it of oxygen and causing it to die. This is called a stroke. The increased risk of blood clots is a result of the atria not emptying properly. Blood that is not moving tends to clot. A stroke means that an area of brain tissue dies from lack of oxygen. This may cause paralysis or weakness in an arm and/or leg or loss of speech or partial visual loss. Clots can also affect the kidneys (causing stomach pains and blood in the urine) or the leg (causing the leg to go white and painful and, if untreated, gangrene).

Treatment of heart failure and atrial fibrillation
Treatment with medicine
For most people with heart failure and atrial fibrillation, treatment consists of medicines to slow the conduction of impulses from the atria to the ventricles (usually a combination of digoxin and beta blockers is required) and medicines to reduce the risk of blood clots. Warfarin is effective. Aspirin is not effective and may make things worse in this situation.

For many patients with atrial fibrillation, the best management is not to try to get the heart back into a normal rhythm, but rather just to stop the heart going too fast and to thin the blood, using the above treatments.

Electric shock treatment (cardioversion)
Treatment with medicines can restore a normal heart rhythm in about one patient in five. Electric shock treatment (electrical cardioversion) can restore a normal rhythm in most patients. This is generally performed in hospital, under a general anaesthetic or heavy sedation. The electric shock disrupts the heart's abnormal electrical rhythm allowing a normal rhythm to take over again in many cases.

Unfortunately, most patients will relapse within a few months. Research has shown that electric shock therapy to restore a normal heart rhythm is associated with a slightly higher risk of stroke, than just controlling the heart rhythm with medicines. Therefore electrical cardioversion is recommended only in selected cases or as part of research studies to try to find safer and more effective methods of cardioversion.

Catheter ablation

Catheter ablation, as performed in 2004 on the British Prime Minister, Tony Blair, is a promising experimental technique for patients with heart failure and atrial fibrillation. It involves passing some small wires from the vein in the leg to the heart. An electric current will then be used to 'microwave' part of the heart to block the abnormal electrical conduction. The procedure is not without risk, including occasional fatalities. It is not for everyone!

Valve disease

The purpose of a heart valve is to allow blood to flow in one direction only. This means that it will let blood into a chamber or major vessel, but won't let it back out the way it came in. There are two ways in which a heart valve can become damaged:

1. It can become narrowed (stenosis), so not enough blood can be pushed through the gap with each beat of the heart; the heart tries to pump harder, putting it under extra strain.

2. It can become leaky or incompetent (regurgitation). In this case, some blood will flow back into the chamber that it came from, so again the heart

Heart valves

There are four heart valves.

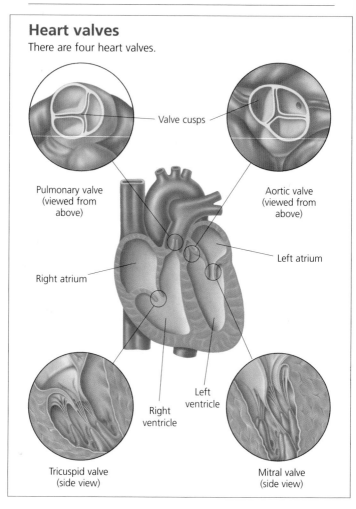

Valve cusps

Pulmonary valve
(viewed from
above)

Aortic valve
(viewed from
above)

Left atrium

Right atrium

Left
ventricle

Right
ventricle

Tricuspid valve
(side view)

Mitral valve
(side view)

needs to work harder to pump enough blood out in
the right direction.

Any of the four heart valves may become diseased,
but the mitral or aortic valves are most often affected.
This is because they are both in the left side of the

Function of heart valves

Heart valves – normal and abnormal function.

Healthy valves   **Diseased valves**

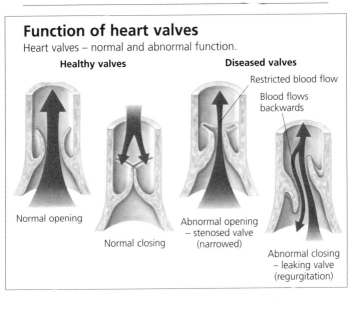

Restricted blood flow

Blood flows backwards

Normal opening

Normal closing

Abnormal opening – stenosed valve (narrowed)

Abnormal closing – leaking valve (regurgitation)

heart which is exposed to much higher pressures and stresses than the right side. Over 99 per cent of heart valve operations are on one or other of these valves.

Older people may have suffered damage to their heart valves as a consequence of having had rheumatic fever in childhood or early adult life, but, fortunately, this is now rare in the developed world. Valves may also be damaged by infections (such as endocarditis – see box on page 30) or by some immune system disorders. Valves may leak or become stiff simply as part of the ageing process. The box lists the most common causes of valvular heart disease (VHD) in terms of stenosis or regurgitation, although it is quite possible to have 'mixed valve disease', that is, a combination of the two.

Sometimes you may be aware that you have a problem with a heart valve before you get any symptoms.

Causes of valve disease

Cause of valvular stenosis	Description
Rheumatic fever	An infection, usually caught in childhood
	Uncommon to get this nowadays, but people who had it many years ago have now become old enough to have the associated heart problems
Calcification	As we get older many tissues in the body get calcium deposits in them, making them harder and less supple. This happens in the heart valves, but is much faster and more severe in some people than others
Congenital	These are defects that we are born with, and are sometimes inherited from our parents' genes
	They may show up immediately after birth, later in life or not at all, depending on their nature and severity

Cause of valvular regurgitation	Description
Rheumatic fever	See above
Ischaemic	After a heart attack, dead areas of heart muscle may involve the cords and tendons that operate the valve, making it leak
Congenital	See above
Floppy valves	Results from degeneration of the valve tissue
Infective (endocarditis)	An infection of a heart valve is extremely serious, and is often a life-threatening emergency
Long-standing high blood pressure	See page 22

This is particularly common if you have a congenital (or inborn) defect which has been picked up by chance or in the course of having tests for some other routine operation. Not everyone who has a diseased heart valve will need an operation. Some people can live happily all their life with no symptoms at all, and others may respond well to medicines.

Many heart valve problems increase the risk of bacteria in the blood settling on the valve, causing infection and damaging the valves further. This is called endocarditis. The bugs get into the blood as a result of either poor oral hygiene or dental work (scaling of the teeth or extractions – that is, anything that causes the gums to bleed). You should ask whether you should take a dose of antibiotics before seeing the dentist or having an operation if you have a heart valve problem.

Heart muscle disease

Some people with poorly functioning heart muscles have normal coronary arteries, excluding coronary disease as a cause of heart failure, and the doctor must look elsewhere for the cause of the damage.

Sometimes, none can be found; this condition is known as dilated cardiomyopathy, meaning that the heart has become large and pumps weakly. Sometimes the problem is genetic, in which case several members of the family will be affected.

There is no doubt that drinking excessive quantities of alcohol (regular heavy drinking over a number of years) poisons the heart muscle and can cause heart failure. It is also possible for cardiomyopathy to be the result of a virus infection.

Hypertrophic cardiomyopathy means that the heart muscle has become thick and stiff. This usually presents with problems other than heart failure (chest pains or heart rhythm problems). It also commonly runs in families.

Overall, heart muscle disease accounts for only about one in fifty of those people with heart failure, but it is responsible for a much higher proportion of cases in young people.

Dyssynchrony

In some patients the heart muscle is pumping fairly well but not in unison. One bit may start pumping before the others, which just puts a strain on the relaxed bits of the heart, causing them to bulge outwards without doing anything useful, such as pumping blood out of the heart. The bit that pumps first also relaxes first, just as the 'late' parts of the heart start to pump. These late bits waste a lot of their energy causing the bit that contracted first to bulge outwards. This problem can be treated with a clever pacemaker (see page 76).

Can other diseases play a part?

People who already have heart failure or who could be at risk after a heart attack should be checked (and treated if possible) for any other illnesses that might bring on heart failure or make it worse. Anaemia and thyroid and kidney problems are the main causes of concern.

Anaemia

The red colour of blood comes from haemoglobin, which is how it carries oxygen. Blood is bright red when saturated with oxygen (arterial blood) and dark red when low in oxygen (venous blood). If the red blood cell count is low (anaemia), the blood is less efficient at carrying oxygen, the most essential 'nutrient' for the body. This means that not only is the heart muscle receiving less oxygen, but it also has to work harder to supply the tissues with all the oxygen that they need. It's easy to see how the additional workload created by the anaemia can put a strain on an already damaged heart and so cause heart failure. Patients with heart failure and anaemia have worse symptoms, more hospitalisations for worsening heart failure and a poor overall outcome.

The reasons for anaemia in heart failure are complex. Sometimes anaemia is the result of a lack of the nutrients required to make haemoglobin (iron, folate and vitamin B_{12}) due either to a poor diet or to bowel disease. The levels of these can be checked in the blood and any deficiency corrected with tablets. If the anaemia is due to iron deficiency then the bowel motions need to be tested for blood. If this test is positive, then further investigations to exclude stomach ulcers and bowel tumours are required.

However, in many cases the anaemia is just another sign of a failing heart. There is growing research evidence that the bone marrow can be stimulated to produce more blood by injecting larger amounts of a substance called erythropoietin than the body itself produces. New synthetic versions of this hormone may require injection only once or twice per month. The safety and efficacy of this treatment are still under investigation, but it looks promising.

Thyroid problems

The thyroid gland produces a hormone that regulates the rate at which most of the body's functions work, including the heart. An over- or under-active gland can cause problems. Anyone who has developed atrial fibrillation should always have a blood test to check whether his or her thyroid is functioning normally.

Kidney problems

The heart and kidneys work closely together, so when one runs into problems it is bound to affect the other. The kidneys are responsible for getting rid of excess water and salt from the body and, when they stop working properly, too much of both of these is retained. Fluid retention will cause weight gain. Clothing or rings may become tighter and the person may develop symptoms such as breathlessness and ankle swelling – which are similar to those caused by heart failure. What's more, having too much fluid in your circulation can put an added strain on the heart. On the other hand, heart failure means that less blood reaches the kidneys, reducing their efficiency so that they can't get rid of fluid properly. In turn, this can make heart failure worse. Kidney problems can be excluded by a simple blood test. Patients with both heart and kidney problems require expert advice and careful management.

The difference between heart disease and heart failure

Just because you have a problem with your heart, it doesn't mean that you are bound to develop heart failure. For example, most people who have angina don't have heart failure. Their main problem is chest pain which usually comes on when they exercise and stops when they rest. It is caused by reduced blood flow to the heart muscle itself.

The term 'heart failure' tells you only that the heart is not working well enough to pump nutrients and oxygen to the tissues – it doesn't tell you why. In fact, as we have seen, there are several possible explanations.

KEY POINTS

■ Heart failure has many causes

■ Different causes of heart disease may require different treatment

Diagnosing heart failure

Spotting the symptoms

Having looked at the way the heart and circulation work, it may be easier to understand why heart failure causes the symptoms that it does.

Breathlessness

Usually, this means feeling short of breath when doing some activity that wouldn't normally cause any problems for someone of a similar age – such as walking up a flight of stairs at your own pace. In most cases, the breathlessness will have got worse over a period of days, weeks or months.

At worst, you may even feel short of breath while resting. However, you must remember that there are many other conditions, such as asthma and chronic bronchitis, that can cause breathlessness, so don't jump to conclusions.

One of the features typical of severe heart failure is needing to sleep propped up in bed, sometimes with five or six pillows. You may find that you wake up feeling very short of breath because you have slipped down in the bed. Sitting upright or getting out of bed will usually ease the breathing after 20 minutes or so, but if it doesn't you should phone your doctor who will probably give you an injection to clear the excess fluid quickly.

Even if your symptoms do settle fairly promptly, waking at night with severe breathlessness means that your heart failure is not well controlled and you should see your doctor very soon.

Breathlessness and heart failure

Breathlessness is a frequently occurring symptom of heart failure.

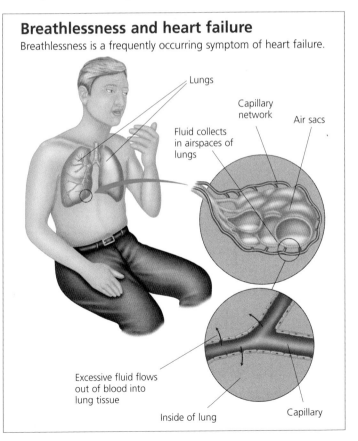

Lungs

Capillary network

Air sacs

Fluid collects in airspaces of lungs

Excessive fluid flows out of blood into lung tissue

Inside of lung

Capillary

The reasons why heart failure causes breathlessness are not fully understood. Increases in the pressure in the capillaries in the lung probably lead to a build-up of fluid in the lung which increases lung stiffness and stops oxygen getting into the blood so easily. If the small airspaces in the lungs fill up with fluid this can make breathing even at rest very difficult.

The reasons why people get breathless on exertion are probably even more complex. In patients with heart failure it may be a combination of a lack of fitness and the illness itself that causes breathlessness on exertion. For this reason, provided that heart failure is not severe, doctors generally recommend regular exercise on a daily basis, which is sufficient to make you breathless without making you feel ill.

Swollen ankles

Many normal, healthy people get mildly swollen ankles at times, for example, in hot weather, after a long journey, before a menstrual period or in pregnancy, or if they have varicose veins. However, increasing ankle swelling may be a symptom of heart failure, in which case it is likely to affect both legs equally. In the same way that heart failure causes fluid in the lungs to collect and cause breathlessness, it can also cause fluid to leak out of blood vessels in the body and collect in the tissues, especially the legs.

The actual cause of the leakage is complicated but, in simple terms, as the pressure in the heart rises, this causes the pressure in the veins to rise. This creates a back pressure that causes fluid to leak from the blood vessels. Fluid collects most commonly in the ankles simply because of the force of gravity. In worsening heart failure, the swelling can creep further up the legs.

Swollen ankles

Swollen ankles can be a symptom of heart failure.

Back pressure in veins, together with gravity, oppose return blood flow in veins

Veins

Fluid accumulates in legs

Red blood cells

Tissues

Swollen ankles

Fluid forced out of capillaries into tissues

Capillary

Pressing your thumb into the swollen area for 30 seconds will leave a dent which takes a minute or so to disappear. Staying in bed may get rid of swelling round the ankles, but the fluid may collect around the lower part of the back instead.

There are other reasons why one leg might suddenly swell up. People who had the veins taken out of one leg, often for a heart bypass operation, are more likely to develop swelling in that leg. If the calf is painful, you should see a doctor immediately because this might be the result of a blood clot in one of the leg veins.

Passing more urine at night

As everyone's kidneys work more efficiently when they're lying down, people with heart failure sometimes notice that they pass more urine during the night. Again, there could be other explanations for this – such as an enlarged prostate in men.

Fatigue

This can be a symptom of virtually any medical problem or a normal response to overdoing things. Everyone feels tired at some time but if you're tired all the time without any obvious reason, you should see your doctor. Fatigue can be a symptom of many diseases, including mental stress, depression and viral infections, as well as of heart failure.

A person with heart failure may feel constantly tired because of the poor supply of oxygen and nutrients and the accumulation of waste products in their muscles.

Remember . . .

Heart failure can be diagnosed only by a doctor after he or she has heard about the symptoms and examined the patient. Tests are always needed to confirm the diagnosis (see below).

Is it heart failure?
How your doctors decide what's wrong

Diagnosing heart failure has to be left to doctors because all the main symptoms can be caused by other illnesses or can sometimes affect normal healthy people. Your symptoms, together with the physical examination, are usually enough to alert your doctor to the possibility of heart failure.

All patients need further tests to confirm the diagnosis and to try to discover its cause. A set of guidelines, drawn up by doctors who are experts on the subject, recommends that anyone with suspected heart failure should have tests.

It is important to detect heart failure as early as possible so that, whenever possible, the underlying problem can be put right or at least treated so that it doesn't get any worse.

A blood test called BNP or NT-proBNP (B-type natriuretic peptide) can help doctors detect heart failure early and monitor its progress. Patients with suspected heart failure who have a normal BNP test almost always turn out to have other reasons for their symptoms. If your pulse is irregular, an ECG will confirm whether or not you have atrial fibrillation. Most patients will have an echocardiogram which is very good at diagnosing 'weak' hearts and valve problems. It is less clear how useful the echocardiogram is in diagnosing heart failure resulting from a 'stiff' heart. The BNP blood test seems to be a better way of diagnosing this, provided that there is no complicating kidney problem. However, patients with heart rhythm problems such as atrial fibrillation (see page 24) often have increased BNP results of a moderate degree, even if heart function is otherwise normal.

The modern 'gold-standard' diagnostic technique is magnetic resonance imaging (MRI), although this is available only in larger hospitals at the moment. MRI is the most accurate way of assessing heart muscle function, can distinguish heart scars (which respond poorly to all current forms of treatment) from 'sleeping' or 'hibernating' heart muscle (which is more likely to respond) and assess valve function. It has been perceived as a very expensive investigation in the past but costs are falling dramatically. It is likely that, in the future, many patients with suspected heart failure will have this test.

Blood tests are always required to detect anaemia and kidney problems.

Checks and tests for suspected heart failure

Most people should have the following basic investigations if heart failure is suspected and some may need further more specialised tests afterwards. We look at all these in more detail in the next few pages.

- Physical examination – this is likely to include taking your pulse and blood pressure, listening to your heart and lungs, checking the veins in your neck and looking for any swelling of legs or lower spine
- Blood test
- Chest X-ray
- ECG (electrocardiogram)
- Echocardiogram.

Physical examination

Check	What?	Why?
Pulse	How fast?	A heart that beats too quickly or too slowly cannot pump efficiently
	Is it regular?	Conditions such as atrial fibrillation which cause irregular heartbeat can lead to heart failure
	Character	Sometimes the feel of the pulse can be a clue to problems such as valve disease
Blood pressure	Too high?	High blood pressure can put a strain on the heart and cause heart failure in the long term
	Too low?	This can cause dizziness, blackouts or kidney problems

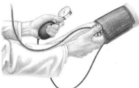

Blood pressure test.

Check	What?	Why?
Heart	How it sounds	Any noises heard between the normal sounds of the valves opening and closing indicate turbulent blood flow from a narrowed or leaky valve
Neck	Vein	When the heart isn't pumping properly, pressure backs up in the veins and the vein in the side of the neck becomes distended
Ankles	Swollen?	Fluid can collect in the lower legs and the lower back and occasionally people with heart failure have swollen stomachs

Blood test

This is to check for anaemia and kidney problems, both of which can make heart failure worse (see pages 32–4). If your heart rhythm is irregular, your blood will also be tested for thyroid hormone levels. An overactive gland can cause atrial fibrillation (see page 33). A normal BNP test makes heart failure very unlikely.

Blood test

A blood test will check for any problems with the kidneys or thyroid and for anaemia.

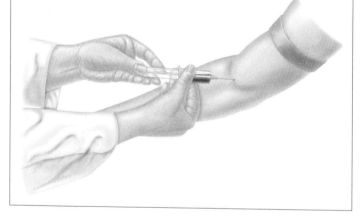

Chest X-ray

This simple and familiar test produces a variety of useful information:

- The size and shape of the heart and whether it has changed, by becoming enlarged, for example
- Whether fluid has collected in the airspaces of the lungs as a result of heart failure
- Whether there is any lung disease causing breathlessness.

Chest X-ray

A chest X-ray will check whether there are problems with the heart and lungs.

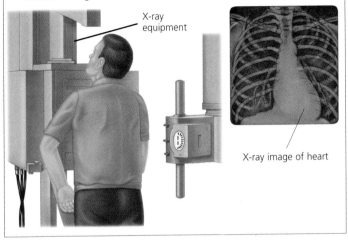

X-ray equipment

X-ray image of heart

ECG (electrocardiogram)

Every time the heart beats, it causes natural electrical changes, and the ECG records this activity in different sites around the body. The electrical signals are picked up through pads attached across the chest and at other points such as ankles or wrists. These ECG traces give the doctor lots of information about the heart, depending on whether and how they differ from the normal patterns. The doctor can assess heart rate and rhythm and whether the heart muscle is conducting electricity normally. Damaged muscle or muscle that is short of oxygen produces a different tracing.

If the problem is intermittent irregular heartbeats, it can be difficult to spot on a simple ECG tracing when the heart may happen to be beating normally. One way of getting round this situation is for the person to wear a

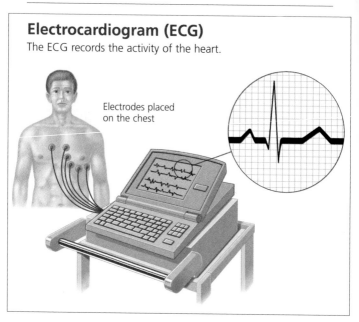

Electrocardiogram (ECG)

The ECG records the activity of the heart.

Electrodes placed on the chest

very small portable ECG machine on a belt or over the shoulder for 24 hours. Any time the person feels any symptoms, he or she presses a button which marks the recording. When the results are analysed later, the symptom marker can be compared with the tracing of the heartbeat at that time. Some machines record a heart tracing that can be transmitted down a telephone line to a doctor for an instant opinion or advice.

Echocardiogram

This test involves bouncing sound waves into the heart from a plastic probe placed on the chest. The technique is much the same as the ultrasound scans used to check unborn babies during pregnancy. It allows the doctor to see how the heart muscle and valves are working. This is particularly useful as the

Echocardiogram

The echocardiogram shows how the heart muscle and valves are working.

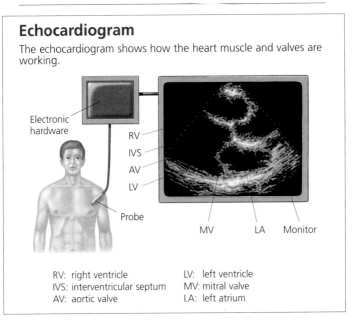

RV: right ventricle
IVS: interventricular septum
AV: aortic valve

LV: left ventricle
MV: mitral valve
LA: left atrium

doctor can actually see the heart beating and check different areas for problems.

Your own doctor may be able to do the blood test and ECG, but the chest X-ray and echocardiogram usually have to be done at a hospital. Depending on the local set-up, you may or may not have to see a heart specialist. Although specialist services are available in most areas of the country, waiting lists are sometimes long. Many hospitals are setting up special clinics to provide an efficient service for people with heart failure, and echocardiography is becoming more widely available.

Further investigations

If the results of these tests show that you could benefit from an operation or other special treatment, you might need some extra tests.

Exercise test

Using a treadmill or bicycle: this helps the specialist to decide how well your heart copes with exercise. Electrodes are placed on your chest and your heart is monitored at varying levels of exercise. You may be asked to breathe into a mask to check how much oxygen the body is using.

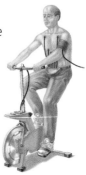

Nuclear heart scan

There are several versions that involve injecting a very small amount of radioactive material into the bloodstream and then using a special camera to measure various aspects of heart function.

Nuclear heart scan

The nuclear heart scan measures various aspects of heart function.

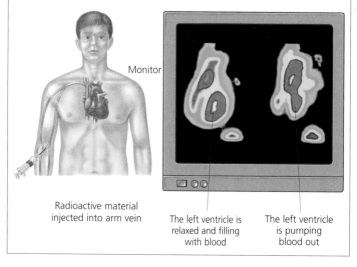

Monitor

Radioactive material injected into arm vein

The left ventricle is relaxed and filling with blood

The left ventricle is pumping blood out

Angiogram

This may be needed if you are having surgery on a valve or a blocked coronary artery. Fine tubes are threaded through blood vessels in your groin or arm under local anaesthetic and threaded up to your heart. Special dye is then injected which allows X-rays to be taken to assess the severity of any problem in the valve or artery and what, if anything, needs to be done to correct it.

Angiogram

An angiogram may be performed if you are to undergo surgery.

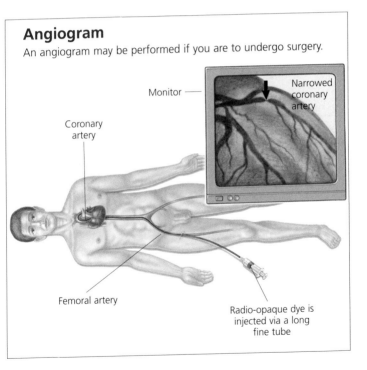

Monitor

Narrowed coronary artery

Coronary artery

Femoral artery

Radio-opaque dye is injected via a long fine tube

Magnetic resonance imaging

Magnetic resonance imaging (MRI) uses powerful magnets to align the subatomic particles in the part of the body being studied. Radiowave pulses break the alignment causing signals to be emitted from the atoms. These signals can be measured and a detailed image built up of the tissues and organs.

Magnetic resonance imaging (MRI)

MRI is used to image the organs and tissues.

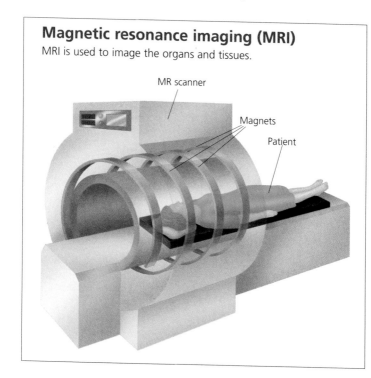

MR scanner

Magnets

Patient

KEY POINTS

Most patients require hospital tests to:

■ Ensure that heart failure is the cause of the symptoms

■ Discover what the cause of the heart failure is

■ Discover if there are other complicating factors

The right treatment

Treatment goals

When treating heart failure, doctors have simple and clear aims in mind:

- To stop things getting worse for as long as possible in a person who feels well
- To help someone who does not feel well to feel better and enable him or her to do more
- To prolong the person's life.

What treatment each person has will depend on his or her condition. Most types of treatment that maintain or improve the way the person feels will also help him or her to live longer. Sometimes, however, treatment that is given to prolong life may have side effects that make people feel worse and these may not be acceptable to some people.

Medical treatment

Usually people with heart failure will need to take pills lifelong to help control symptoms and delay or stop progression of the underlying heart problem. Some may benefit from pacemakers or surgery.

As we have seen, heart failure can sometimes be the result of another underlying illness such as anaemia, or thyroid or kidney disease, so the first step is to correct any such problem if at all possible. For some people, this may be all the treatment that is needed. For most people with heart failure, however, regular, long-term medicines will be needed to help the heart function as near normally as possible.

Medical treatment is a very complex subject with a large number of medicines on the market. The matter is further complicated by the fact that the pharmaceutical companies all give their products 'proprietary/trade' names as well as their actual 'generic/scientific' name.

Consequently, if one medicine is manufactured by three different companies, it will have three different names. This can be confusing because you may be on exactly the same medication as somebody you know, but you each have different names on the boxes of your tablets! Occasionally two medicines are combined in a single tablet.

Medical treatment for some forms of heart failure is not always effective. For example, there is less evidence that treatment of 'stiff' hearts does any good. In such cases, good control of high blood pressure, atrial fibrillation and fluid retention is often effective. Heart failure caused by narrowed or leaking valves needs evaluation by a cardiologist to determine whether surgery will help.

The following section concentrates mainly on patients with heart failure caused by a 'weak heart' but also deals with 'confused hearts' (the two sorts of problem often coexist).

Treatments mainly directed at heart failure caused by a weak heart

Almost all doctors agree that all patients with a weak heart should be treated with an angiotensin-converting enzyme inhibitor and a beta blocker, unless they do not tolerate the treatment or there are special reasons why they cannot take them.

Most experts will add a third treatment, although opinion is split between whether this should be an angiotensin receptor blocker (ARB) or an aldosterone antagonist. Some experts would give all four. In addition most patients will need a diuretic to treat fluid retention and many will receive other treatments for underlying coronary disease.

The effects of each of these treatments is relatively small but the combined effects of these treatments, in terms of improved symptoms, reduced admission to hospital and prolongation of life, is large.

ACE inhibitors
How they work

Angiotensin-converting enzyme (ACE) is a chemical produced naturally by the body. Its task is to make another chemical, called angiotensin, and this is responsible for constricting blood vessels and making the kidneys retain salt and water.

Normally, angiotensin is produced in response to some problem with the circulation – such as a large loss of blood or heart failure. Production of angiotensin as a result of heart failure becomes a vicious circle whereby blood vessels become more constricted, increasing the pressure on the heart, which causes the body to produce more angiotensin, and so on.

will cause the blood pres
usually allow a weight ga
kilograms (two to four p
medical advice). You sho
of the ACE inhibitor exce

Coughing is common
even when they aren't ta
caused by the medicine i
persistent, and may well
from sleeping. If the cou
blocker (see below) may

Kidney problems som
some people to take AC
treatment can cause bot
and excessive increases i
which can make people
the heart. Other patient
able to take ACE inhibit
come off other blood pr
water tablets, or can tak
doses. If you have kidne
keep a close eye on you

Angiotensin recepto

These agents block the
opposed to the effect o
reduce the production o
advantage of not causin
Recent research sugges
inhibitors and angioten
symptoms, reduce prob
hospital and possibly pi
able to advise you whe

ACE inhibitors work by interrupting this cycle, reducing the production of a hormone called angiotensin II. In so doing, they relieve breathlessness and enable the person to be more active. They also delay or prevent any further deterioration in heart function, helping people with heart failure to live longer.

They need to be taken together with water tablets if the person has fluid retention – swollen ankles, for example (see page 60).

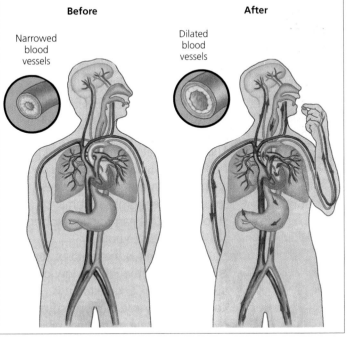

How ACE inhibitors work

Constricted blood vessels raise blood pressure and make the heart work harder. Use of ACE inhibitors opens up blood vessels, resulting in a reduction in blood pressure and in the workload of the heart.

Before

After

Narrowed blood vessels

Dilated blood vessels

As well as being
inhibitors may also |
or to protect the he
reduce the risk of h
problems from dev(

Side effects

As with any medici
side effects when t
mostly minor and (
weeks. Headaches
common. More tro
dizziness and coug
with a bit of help.

Dizziness is caus
veins and arteries r
trigger a blackout if
to get blood up to
likely to happen to
she has been takin
tablets) for some ti
to lie down after t(
for a few hours an

Anyone who is k
be asked to take tl
of a doctor or nurs
becomes a persiste
require investigatio
or a narrowing in 1

If the blood pre
heart failure and it
pressure may be c(
usually best to try
This allows the bo(

to be taught to avoid them in patients with heart failure. Research has now shown that, started in very small doses and increased very slowly, they may be remarkably effective in reducing symptoms, strengthening the heart (in the long term) and helping people with heart failure stay out of hospital and live longer.

At the moment, experts disagree about whether this beneficial effect applies to all beta blockers or just to certain ones, such as bisoprolol, carvedilol and nebivolol. There is also controversy about whether these three beta blockers are equally effective.

Side effects

Side effects are not uncommon when starting a beta blocker. They can cause the airways to get narrower, which can be dangerous in people with asthma. Dizziness, fatigue and increased breathlessness may be encountered. Patients with diabetes may notice that their blood sugar tends to run higher, although they seem to get greater long-term benefit. With time, side effects usually resolve and after two to three months the benefits of beta blockers begin to appear. Some patients can respond dramatically but often it takes time! In a few cases, beta blockers may even cure heart failure. Patience is required.

The doses of beta blocker should be increased gradually at two- to four-weekly intervals over a period of months to achieve maintenance doses. Increasing the dose more quickly often leads to problems.

Beta blockers may also be used, along with digoxin, to control atrial fibrillation.

Water tablets (or diuretics)
How they work
Diurectics force the kidneys to get rid of salt and water.

This lowers blood pressure by reducing the volume of liquid in the circulation thus reducing the pressure in the blood vessels. As a result, they can help with symptoms such as breathlessness and swollen ankles, which result from waterlogging of the tissues; however, they don't have any effect on other problems associated with heart failure as far as we know.

They are often prescribed for people whose heart failure is newly diagnosed because they work quickly and can do only good in the short term, whatever the cause of the heart failure.

Your GP can get you to start taking them to relieve breathlessness and swollen ankles while investigations are being organised to find out what is the root cause of your symptoms – in other words, to confirm that you do have heart failure and if so why. Once you have a detailed diagnosis, other treatments can be prescribed if you need them.

The amount of urine you pass or the quantity of fluid that you retain can cause measurable changes in your weight. Each litre of urine weighs one kilogram (2.2 pounds). By weighing yourself every day at the same time and in the same clothes (for example, in the morning wearing pyjamas), you can check the amount of water you're passing out of the body in your urine. If you find that you have gained more than two to three kilograms (four to six pounds) in one week and you are also becoming short of breath, you should ask your doctor whether you need to increase your dose of water tablets. If you can't get to speak to him or her, take an extra tablet and talk to the doctor the following day. Once you get more experienced, you may be able to control how many water tablets you need to take by yourself.

How diuretics affect the body

Diuretics help the kidneys to get rid of salt and water in the urine, reducing the volume of circulating blood, thus reducing pressure in the circulation.

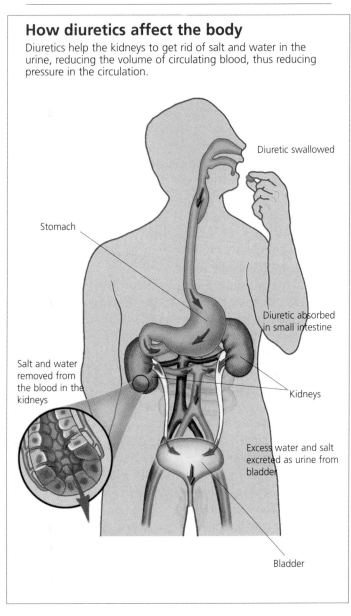

Diuretic swallowed

Stomach

Diuretic absorbed in small intestine

Salt and water removed from the blood in the kidneys

Kidneys

Excess water and salt excreted as urine from bladder

Bladder

On the other hand, an attack of diarrhoea that leaves you two to three kilograms lighter probably means that you should cut out the water tablets for a few days until your weight is back to normal. Don't hesitate to ask your doctor's or nurse's advice in situations like this – usually a brief telephone call will be enough to answer all your questions.

Side effects

Anyone who is taking powerful water tablets for the first time should bear in mind that you need to have easy access to a toilet for a few hours after your first dose. Usually, the amount of urine will be less dramatic after the first few doses, but it's a good idea to take them at least four to six hours before bedtime so you don't have to get up during the night.

Should you have to be somewhere where you can't be sure of getting to a toilet easily, it is worth postponing taking the water tablet until a more convenient time of day.

One important possible side effect of the more powerful diuretics is urinary retention in those men whose prostate gland is enlarged. The kidneys are stimulated by the tablets into producing urine much faster than usual, causing the bladder to overfill. It is important to tell or remind your doctor if you have difficulty passing urine or any problem with bladder control before you take any new water tablets.

Some people develop gout as a result of taking water tablets – the main symptom is usually a hot and painful big toe. This can be treated and subsequent attacks prevented by adding an anti-gout medicine.

Gout is caused by uric acid in the following way: uric acid is a normal waste product of the body's metabolism and is filtered into the urine by the kidneys. Diuretics reduce the amount of uric acid passed out in the urine. This causes uric acid levels to rise in the blood and tissues, When the levels are high enough it crystallises out in the joints causing gout pain.

You're likely to have regular blood tests several times a year to check for any sign that your kidneys are working less efficiently (if this happens you may need to have your tablets changed). If you're on ACE inhibitors as well as water tablets, dizziness is a possible side effect. If you do experience this, talk to your doctor who will probably reduce the dose of diuretics.

Most diuretics cause the body to lose a substance called potassium and this can lead to a feeling of weakness and rhythm upsets in the heart. Other diuretics can help the body hold on to potassium. These include aldosterone antagonists (spironolactone and eplerenone) (see page 57). Potassium-losing and -retaining diuretics are often given together to keep the potassium balance right. In some patients with severe heart failure, other types of diuretics may be used for additional effect – some of these can make you pass an awful lot of urine.

Digoxin

How it works

This is the purified form of digitalis, which was made for centuries from foxgloves. Treatment in tablet form is rather more reliable than the old herbal preparations, which poisoned many people. Although digoxin in its natural form was discovered by an Englishman called William Withering over 200 years ago, we still don't really know how it works or how useful it really is.

Popular tradition suggests that it strengthens weakened heart muscle, but we don't know whether this is really an important part of its action. It is certainly effective at controlling the heart rate, which is why it is a popular choice for treating people whose heart failure is caused by atrial fibrillation.

Doctors disagree about whether digoxin should be prescribed for people whose heart rhythm is regular – some think it should be reserved only for particularly difficult cases. Digoxin may improve symptoms in some patients in this setting but has little or no effect on hospitalisation or longevity in studies conducted to date.

Side effects

Of all the tablets prescribed for heart failure, digoxin is probably the one with the fewest side effects when taken in the appropriate dose, but if it builds up in the body it can be dangerous. The kidneys get rid of it very slowly. Once you stop taking it, it will be about a week before all traces of it disappear from your system.

Older people (aged 75 years or over) and anyone with kidney problems can take digoxin only in small doses. Too much of it may provoke feelings of nausea and vomiting, and some people start seeing everything tinged with yellow; older people may become confused. Anyone who suspects that he or she has developed any of these side effects should stop taking digoxin immediately and contact his or her doctor for advice.

Nitrates

Nitrates work by relaxing the blood vessels, both arteries and veins. These medicines are frequently taken by people with angina (caused by lack of adequate blood supply to the heart muscle). It is unclear whether they are really useful for patients with heart failure, except for the treatment of severe breathlessness at rest –

How heart medicines can be given

There are many different categories of heart medicines and they can be given in a variety of ways.

Sublingually:
Tablet is placed under the tongue until it dissolves

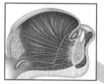

Buccally:
Held between the upper gum and lip while it dissolves

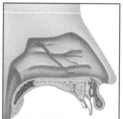

Aerosol spray:
Directed into the mouth

Swallowed:
As tablets or capsules

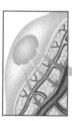

Self-adhesive patch:
The medicine in the patch is absorbed through skin directly into the bloodstream

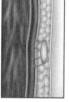

Subcutaneously:
Injected underneath the skin

Intravenously: Rapidly injected directly into a vein or more slowly through an intravenous drip
Intramuscularly: Injection deep into a muscle mass, for example, the buttocks

How nitrates work

Nitrates work by relaxing the arteries and veins, so improving the blood flow in the coronary arteries.

Before nitrate
Constricted coronary artery

After nitrate
Dilated coronary artery

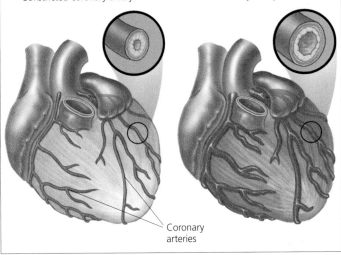

Coronary arteries

when it is usually given intravenously. Nitrate tablets probably do help some people. The patient or doctor, however, may wish to try and see if it makes a difference in his or her situation.

Nitrates, for angina, can be taken in several different ways:

- as a spray used under the tongue
- as tablets to be dissolved between the gums and cheek.

They are also available as skin patches. The medicine is in the patch, which looks like transparent plaster, and is absorbed through the skin into the circulation.

The medicine does not work directly on the heart so there is no advantage in putting the patch on the skin over your heart, but some people like the idea!

Aspirin and anti-platelet agents

These agents (aspirin, clopidogrel and dipyridamole) reduce the stickiness of cell fragments in the blood called platelets, which are partly responsible for starting the formation of blood clots in arteries.

Unfortunately aspirin also blocks the production of substances in the blood vessel wall that are designed to stop clotting and relax blood vessels. Anti-platelet agents are widely used to try to prevent heart attacks and strokes, although their effectiveness is questionable.

Patients with heart failure taking aspirin are more likely to end up needing to be admitted to hospital for worsening heart failure than those who do not. Some experts in heart failure recommend that aspirin should not be given to patients with heart failure, although many doctors believe that the evidence of harm is not strong enough to make such a recommendation.

Aspirin can irritate the lining of the stomach, making it more likely to bleed and making the risks in patients with heart failure higher. It may be responsible for a substantial proportion of the anaemia associated with heart failure, and it also interferes with warfarin in the circulation and can result in the blood becoming too thin. You should double check with your doctor before taking aspirin and warfarin together.

Clopidogrel may be safer than aspirin but is more expensive. Dipyridamole is untested in patients with heart failure. None of these anti-platelet agents has been shown to be more effective than not giving one at all.

Anticoagulants

These agents (warfarin and heparin) stop blood clots forming in arteries, veins and inside the heart itself. They reduce the risk of stroke in patients with atrial fibrillation by reducing blood clots in the atria. They can also reduce the risk of blood clots that can cause damage to the lung (called a pulmonary embolus) or to the blood supply of the legs or kidneys. However, it is not entirely clear whether they are useful in patients with a regular heart rhythm and therefore most patients with a normal heart rhythm will not be given these treatments.

Warfarin can be given by mouth but heparin is given only by injection and is usually reserved for people admitted to hospital who need treatment quickly.

Warfarin requires regular blood tests (at least every two months and often every few weeks) to ensure that enough is given but not too much: too little and blood clots will not be prevented; too much and the risk of serious bleeding is increased. Warfarin is long acting and it takes days for changes in dose to correct clotting problems. The effects of too much warfarin may be corrected with an injection of vitamin K. The effects of warfarin are influenced by other medicines, especially antibiotics, which can increase the effects of warfarin.

Unless there are very good reasons, all patients with heart failure and atrial fibrillation should receive warfarin. It is not clear whether warfarin is useful for patients with heart failure in a normal heart rhythm. Unlike aspirin, it is not associated with an increased risk of hospital admissions for worsening heart failure.

If you're taking warfarin, you will need regular blood tests to make sure that you are on the correct dose. Warfarin interacts with many other medicines, so you should always remind any doctor you see that you are taking it. You also have to be careful about over-the-counter medicines, especially aspirin, painkillers and treatments for arthritis – ask for advice from your doctor or the pharmacist before taking anything new. If you enjoy alcohol, keep your consumption to sensible levels and avoid binge drinking. Warfarin is broken down in the liver. Alcohol increases the rate at which warfarin is broken down in the liver by speeding up the liver enzymes. If the amount of alcohol you drink varies widely so will the clotting ability of your blood.

Amiodarone

This medicine is often an effective way of controlling abnormal heart rhythms and can sometimes restore a regular rhythm to those with atrial fibrillation, when other treatments haven't worked.

Unfortunately, some people can't take it because of side effects. The most common is sensitisation to sunlight, which is a particular problem for people with fair skins. It can take up to a year for the problem to develop, so it's important to take care when in the sun and ask your doctor for advice immediately if you are at all concerned.

It is also possible for it to cause the thyroid gland to become overactive, so, if you start losing weight rapidly, a sign of thyroid overactivity, while on amiodarone, see your doctor who will arrange a blood test.

Serious side effects can occur in the liver and lungs. Amiodarone can cause jaundice and shortness of breath as a result of lung damage, but these side effects are rare in people taking less than 400 milligrams a day for several years.

For those people who don't experience these side effects, however, amiodarone can be a very effective treatment to keep the heart rhythm regular. However, you must have a detailed medical assessment at least once a year and should ask your doctor whether it is wise to continue.

Calcium channel blockers
How they work
People who have angina or high blood pressure may be treated with calcium channel blockers. These medicines block the action of calcium on the heart muscle and blood vessels. Calcium entering a muscle cell causes it to contract. Calcium channel blockers reduce the amount of calcium entering the muscle cells of the coronary arteries and other blood vessels in the circulation, causing them to relax and get wider. This increases the blood supply to the heart and reduces the work the heart has to do to pump blood round the circulatory system. These are good effects in treating angina and high blood pressure.

Side effects
However, a possible side effect is that the heart may pump less powerfully, making the heart failure worse and causing the body to retain more salt and water. Therefore these medicines are **not** used routinely for heart failure.

Newer calcium channel blockers, such as amlodipine, seem to be safer and may be used in patients with heart failure to treat angina or high blood pressure when other treatments (such as ACE inhibitors, angiotensin receptor blockers and beta blockers and aldosterone antagonists in combination) are not enough.

New medications

Before new medications can become available for use, their value and safety have to be proved before their use is widely recommended. This is achieved through clinical research trials.

Cholesterol-lowering medicines

These days, doctors usually use statins (for example, simvastatin, pravastatin, atorvastatin and rosuvastatin) and more rarely fibrates (for example, bezafibrate and gemfibrozil). Sometimes they will add a drug called ezetimibe for greater effect. There is powerful evidence that statins reduce the risk of heart attack and stroke but less good evidence with the other types of cholesterol-lowering medication. Safety and efficacy of fibrates and ezetimibe in patients with heart failure are unknown. The statin rosuvastatin has recently been investigated. Overall the study was neutral but did suggest that rosuvastatin was safe. There had been worries about the safety of statins in patients with heart failure before this. Closer examination of the studies suggests that, in patients with milder degrees of heart failure, rosuvastatin was rather effective at reducing the risk of further heart attacks and prolonging survival. In patients with more severe problems it didn't seem to make much difference one way or the other.

Many new compounds are being developed that block chemical messengers other than angiotensin (see 'ACE inhibitors', page 54). Whether or not these will produce useful benefits for patients awaits further research.

Devices
External (not requiring anything to be put inside the body)
Cardioversion

This is the medical term for correcting an abnormal heart rhythm using an electric shock. It is always done in hospital, either under a general anaesthetic or, less often, under heavy sedation. It is used in some emergency situations in hospital and as a planned procedure for atrial fibrillation, which is discussed on page 26.

However, recent research suggests that cardioversion is not a great option for many patients with atrial fibrillation. It is reserved for carefully selected patients. Research into appropriate selection and management of patients who might benefit from cardioversion continues.

If you have been on warfarin before cardioversion it should probably be continued life-long even if a normal rhythm is restored.

Enhanced external counter-pulsation (EECP)

This treatment is used predominantly for patients who also have angina. EECP requires a course of 30 to 40 one-hour sessions of treatment usually on separate days in a hospital clinic. The treatment involves strapping 'bags' to the buttocks, thighs and calves. The bags pulsate with each heartbeat, inflating when the heart relaxes and deflating when the heart pumps. This improves the blood supply to the heart and allows it to work more easily. With repeated treatments it appears that the blood supply to the heart improves, reducing or curing angina and possibly strengthening the heart.

Haemofiltration

This treatment is a bit like kidney dialysis. It is designed to remove salt and water from the body by 'washing' the blood through an exchanger. Its use is still experimental. It may be the only way of treating patients with severe heart failure if they do not respond to water pills.

Internal or implanted (requiring some form of operation)

Pacemakers

The muscle of the heart is stimulated to contract by a complex 'wiring' system. When the heart is badly damaged the electrical conduction system within the heart, which controls and triggers heart muscle contraction, may also be damaged, leading to heart 'block' and this may lead to the heart going too slowly.

The patient may notice a worsening of heart failure or blackouts if this happens. A pacemaker can do much the same job as the heart's own wiring system, although never quite as well.

A pacemaker consists of an electronic device and a battery about the size of a matchbox (the battery life is usually many years), which can be inserted under the skin with a small operation, usually under a local anaesthetic. Wires can then be attached to the battery and threaded through the veins to stimulate the heart.

More recently it has been realised that damage to the heart's own wiring system may lead some parts of the surviving heart muscle to contract when other parts relax. This lack of synchrony (synchrony means that all the parts of the heart are contracting together as a 'team') leads to a further loss of the efficiency of the heart. Ordinary pacemakers may make this worse.

Pacemaker surgery

A pacemaker consists of an electronic device and battery which are inserted under the skin. The pacemaker helps the heart beat regularly and at an appropriate rate.

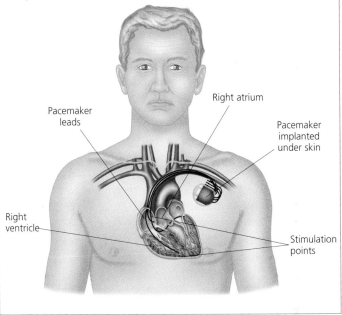

Right atrium

Pacemaker leads

Pacemaker implanted under skin

Right ventricle

Stimulation points

A device similar to a pacemaker can be used to stimulate the heart in a synchronous (coordinated) fashion, increasing its efficiency. This has been shown to improve heart function dramatically in some patients.

In carefully selected patients, these 'cardiac resynchronisation devices' produce marked improvement in symptoms, which helps people with heart failure stay out of hospital and live longer. Perhaps one in four patients with moderate or severe symptoms is suitable for this highly effective treatment.

Implantable defibrillators

Some patients may have serious upsets of their heart rhythm that may cause blackouts or indicate that there is a high risk of the heart stopping. A defibrillator is like a pacemaker (but a little larger) which can give the heart an electric shock if a serious rhythm upset occurs (similar to a cardioversion for atrial fibrillation – see above). These devices are available only in specialist centres. Patients require intensive investigation by a specialist to ascertain whether they are suitable for such treatment. Currently, defibrillators are recommended mostly in patients whose hearts have stopped or almost stopped. It is not clear whether other patients obtain substantial benefit with these devices.

Surgical treatment

If the problem with the heart is structural – a leaky valve or blocked blood vessel, for example – surgery may be possible. For a more complete explanation of surgical treatments see the Family Doctor Book *Understanding Heart Surgery.*

Faulty valves

If the valve is too narrow, or is leaking badly, it will have to be repaired or replaced. Doctors are working on experimental techniques to try to open up narrowed valves or repair leaking ones using various types of keyhole surgery. These are experimental and available in only a few heart centres.

Replacement valves are of two main types: either synthetic, made of metal and plastic, or biological, usually taken from pigs. These days valve surgery is commonplace and, although it is still a major operation,

Valve surgery

In this figure the aortic valve is being replaced with a mechanical valve.

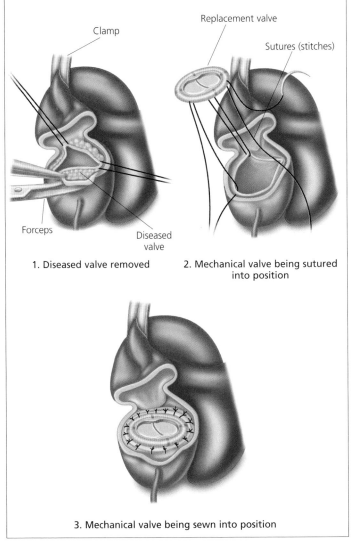

1. Diseased valve removed

2. Mechanical valve being sutured into position

3. Mechanical valve being sewn into position

the success rates are good, provided that patients are well selected and the operation done by an expert.

Narrowed blood vessels

Narrowed blood vessels to the heart muscle may cause angina and heart attacks. It used to be thought that a heart attack always destroyed heart muscle, leaving behind a scar. Recently, it has become clear that heart attacks may just stun heart muscle or put the muscle into a long-term sleep (termed 'hibernation'). Medical treatment, especially beta blockers, or a procedure to improve the blood supply to the heart may revive sleeping (hibernating) heart muscle. Experts disagree about whether pills or one of the procedures below is the safest and most effective way to treat this problem. Preliminary information from the first research study on this topic suggests that medical treatment is satisfactory in most cases but a much larger study should report in the next few years.

Coronary artery bypass graft (CABG)

When coronary arteries (which are the vessels supplying blood to the heart muscle) are blocked or narrowed, too little blood may reach the heart muscle, which stops it contracting properly. In this situation, a coronary bypass operation may be needed. This restores a normal blood supply usually by using a vein from the leg to bypass the blocked sections of coronary artery. Coronary bypass grafting is a major operation, but thousands of people benefit from it every year. Most only have to stay in hospital for a week or 10 days.

For carefully selected patients CABG usually improves angina and sometimes improves breathing problems.

Coronary artery bypass graft

Coronary artery bypass graft – in this figure three vein grafts have been performed (triple bypass).

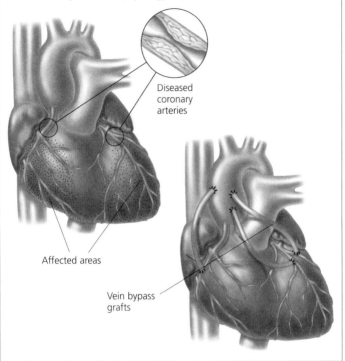

Diseased coronary arteries

Affected areas

Vein bypass grafts

Angioplasty

Sometimes, a narrowed artery can be opened by a procedure called angioplasty, usually combined with a stent (a sort of expandable tubular wire mesh). This involves passing a narrow tube (called a catheter) into the obstructed artery. Around the catheter is a small balloon which is expanded in the narrowed area. It clears the obstruction, opening up the artery so that blood can flow through it properly. The stent holds it open.

Angioplasty

A small balloon is expanded in the narrowed artery to try to open up the artery.

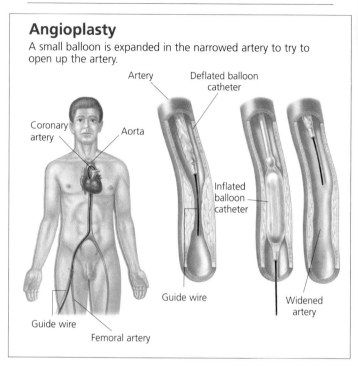

Artery

Deflated balloon catheter

Coronary artery

Aorta

Inflated balloon catheter

Guide wire

Widened artery

Guide wire

Femoral artery

Angioplasty is not suitable for everyone with narrowed blood vessels (angioplasty is less successful if there are multiple blockages), and thorough investigations including catheter tests and heart scans are necessary before the decision is made to use it. There is no evidence that angioplasty reduces the risk of further heart attacks or prolongs life except when used to treat heart attack in the first few hours after the onset of chest pain.

Angioplasty and stenting

A small balloon is inflated in the narrowed artery, the balloon is surrounded by a wire mesh (stent) which also expands and is left in place, when the balloon is withdrawn, to hold the artery open.

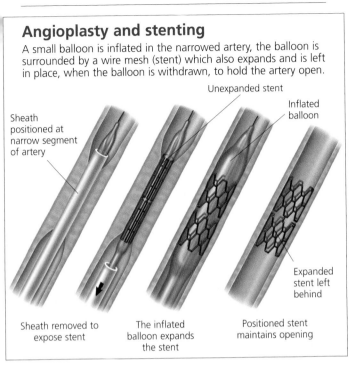

Sheath positioned at narrow segment of artery

Unexpanded stent

Inflated balloon

Expanded stent left behind

Sheath removed to expose stent

The inflated balloon expands the stent

Positioned stent maintains opening

Aneurysmectomy

This procedure involves removing the healed scar from the heart muscle after a severe heart attack, in the hope that this will improve the heart's efficiency. In carefully selected patients this can be quite successful.

Transplantation

This may be an option for younger people with severe heart failure. It is often less useful for people over the age of 60 or so, because they may well have widespread artery disease that makes surgery complicated and means they do less well in the long term. The operation does involve risk, but around 85 per cent of people survive the first month after surgery, and 75 per cent will still be alive five years later.

After surgery, patients who undergo transplantation have to take powerful medicines to prevent their immune systems from rejecting their new heart. As a result of this immune suppression, they are prone to serious infections.

They also need regular tests and biopsies (a technique for picking off a small piece of heart muscle) to check that their new hearts are working properly. Although heart transplantation can be very successful for the right person, it is not a cure.

For many people with mild heart failure, medical treatment is better than a transplantation. In any case, the number of transplantations possible is severely limited by the number of donor hearts available. Around 300 transplantations were done in the UK in 2007. More than 100,000 people developed heart failure over the same period.

Left ventricular assist devices and total artificial hearts

Mechanical devices that can be implanted inside the chest to replace or support heart function have been in development for about 50 years and have achieved some remarkable but not widely publicised success. Hundreds of patients have been kept alive at home with a reasonable quality of life, and sometimes still at work for three or more years, by these devices.

The longest survival time is more than six years. It seems likely that the survival of patients with left ventricular assist devices (LVADs) will exceed the average survival of patients with a biological (human) heart transplant within the next decade.

The best results have been achieved by leaving the 'old' heart in place and using these devices as booster pumps. This has (rarely) even led to recovery of the patient's heart so that the device can be taken out.

Complications include infection and blood clots but these problems can be minimized by careful patient selection and good treatment.

Total artificial hearts are more prone to infection and blood clots and, if they break down, there is no back-up because the 'old' heart has been removed.

Treatment of heart failure caused by stiff hearts

There are no well-proven treatments for heart failure caused by a stiff heart. Doctors will generally treat this problem with water pills. If high blood pressure or atrial fibrillation is present, this will be treated also. There is weak experimental evidence for benefit from beta blockers, aldosterone antagonists or ACE inhibitors.

Telehealth

Careful monitoring of your heart condition can spot problems early and can help ensure that you are on the right doses of medicines. However, most people don't have the luxury of a doctor or nurse who can visit every day. Recently, the National Health Service has begun to implement telemonitoring, which can be done by a telephone link or via a set-top box and a television. This allows patients to record their symptoms, blood pressure, heart rate and rhythm, and in the future many other measures of the heart's health once or twice a day. In my experience most people are willing to spend five minutes twice a day looking after their health when they have a serious condition such

A glossary of hormones related to heart failure

Adenosine	Adenosine is widespread in the body. In the kid it seems responsible for salt and water retention and it may also impair kidney function. Medicin to block these effects are being developed and appear promising
Aldosterone	This hormone is responsible for salt and to a les extent water retention. It does so at the expens of the body losing potassium. Low potassium lev may increase the risk of heart rhythm problems. Salt retention will cause ankle swelling and breathlessness. Aldosterone blockers are widely used in patients with heart failure
Angiotensin II	This hormone is a powerful constrictor of blood vessels. Angiotensin-converting enzyme (ACE) inhibitors reduce its production and angiotensin receptor blockers block its effects
Antidiuretic hormone (otherwise known as Vasopressin)	This hormone stimulates the body to retain wate (but not salt). It may cause the blood sodium to drop and almost certainly contributes to the development of ankle swelling. Medicines to counteract its effects are being developed and may be available within the next few years
Endothelin	Endothelin is a powerful constrictor of blood vessels. Research shows that some special types heart failure caused by very high pressures in th lung (pulmonary hypertension) may benefit from endothelin antagonists. However, large studies c people with the more usual types of heart failur have shown no benefit
Natriuretic peptides	There is a whole family of these peptides, most which are produced by the heart in response to stress. These stimulate the kidney to lose salt an consequently some water. They also tend to rela blood vessels. Increases in this hormone in patie with heart failure should be beneficial. It is probably true that natriuretic peptides delay the development of heart failure and, when this compensatory response is overridden, then hear failure develops. Blood measurements of this hormone can be used to diagnose heart failure and assess its severity

adrenaline adrenaline	These hormones are part of the sympathetic nervous system that, along with the parasympathetic nervous system, forms what is called the autonomic nervous system. The autonomic nervous system is not directly under conscious control but is responsible for a lot of the automatic functions of the body. Noradrenaline and adrenaline are responsible for what is sometimes called the 'fight and flight' response which may cause the heart rate and cardiac output to increase in situations of fear, excitement or exercise. Excess activity may damage the heart and cause rhythm problems. Beta blockers are designed to block these responses. Less is known about the parasympathetic nervous system. Activity seems to be low in heart failure and devices are being developed to try to increase it. Increased parasympathetic activity may reduce heart rhythm problems
staglandins	There is a whole family of prostaglandins in the body. Some, like prostacyclin, are helpful and cause relaxation of blood vessels, improve kidney function and reduce platelet stickiness. Levels are increased in heart failure, rather like the natriuretic peptides, and it may well be that the onset of heart failure reflects the inability of this compensatory response to maintain salt and water balance. Other parts of this system, such as thromboxane, increase platelet stickiness. This may predispose to problems such as a heart attack or stroke. The problem with aspirin in heart failure is that it blocks both good and bad components of this system, which is why other ways of reducing platelet stickiness may be advisable
in	Renin is a hormone produced by the kidney which generates another hormone called angiotensin I that, in turn, is acted on by ACE to produce angiotensin II. A new drug has been developed that blocks renin. Preliminary studies suggest that blocking both renin and ACE at the same time may be beneficial. Further results are awaited

as heart failure. In fact, many patients feel that they are in much more control of the situation when they are making an active contribution. More modern systems give the person with heart failure daily feedback on how they are doing. In fact, it is possible that, in the future, given the growing number of people with heart failure and the limited health resources available, this may be the only way of ensuring continued high-quality care. Of course this will allow people with heart failure to get much more involved in what is going on with their health.

Research studies so far have shown that telemonitoring can ensure that when somebody needs urgent medical attention it can be spotted early. Also, if a patient who has telemonitoring is admitted to hospital, the doctors and nurses are generally happier to let the patient home early because they know that he or she can continue to be monitored at home. Telemonitoring increases life expectancy and the effects seem quite substantial. Many patients like it because it gives them quick access to medical and nursing advice and assistance, when needed.

More recently researchers have added monitoring devices to pacemakers and defibrillators so that these devices can automatically monitor the heart's function. Looking even further into the future, little 'chips' are being developed that can be injected into the body to monitor heart function more or less continuously. For somebody with a severe symptomatic problem, such as heart failure, these monitoring technologies may make all the treatments discussed before work even better.

KEY POINTS

- Most patients require treatment with ACE inhibitors, beta blockers and diuretics and either an aldosterone or angiotensin receptor blocker

- If atrial fibrillation is present, most patients also require digoxin and warfarin

- Experts recommend that you have a thorough review of your medication, together with repeat blood tests to make sure it is not causing a problem, every three to six months; you should arrange this with your doctor

How to help yourself

Although you may depend on your regular medicines to keep you feeling well and active, there is plenty that you can do to help yourself and maximise the benefit that you get from your treatment. Some of the lifestyle changes suggested here may seem difficult, especially at first, but the rewards will come in a greater sense of well-being and important health benefits.

Ways to boost your well-being
Stop smoking
Anyone who smokes already knows that it is bad for the health, but people with heart failure are taking serious extra risks by continuing to smoke:

- It makes it more likely that you will have a (or another) heart attack, so damaging the heart muscle more and making heart failure worse. It makes the blood stickier and promotes the build-up of cholesterol. If you give up smoking after having a heart attack, you greatly reduce your chances of having another one.

- Smokers have lower levels of oxygen in their blood than non-smokers and, as we've seen, diminished oxygen supply to the heart and body is already a problem for people with heart failure. Smoking also causes progressive damage to the lungs.

- The more you smoke the worse it is but even one cigarette constricts the blood vessels, including those in the heart, for 18 hours! The best solution is to give up smoking completely.

Diet

Most patients with heart failure are overweight but some are underweight. People with heart failure appear to do best if well 'nourished'. Loss of muscle bulk or excessive loss of fat is not good.

However, excessive weight does put an extra strain on your heart. People who are seriously overweight should go on a weight-reducing diet. People who are a little overweight should not worry and do not need a weight-reducing diet.

Some people may be overweight because they have retained a lot of fluid. If you are concerned that this may be the case, do not try to work it out for yourself, ask your doctor or a practice nurse. They can give you advice on your target weight and the most sensible way to set about reaching it. There is no evidence that the ideal weight for a healthy person is ideal for people with heart failure; the advice is to attain a body mass index (BMI) between 25 and 29.9 (see page 95).

It is a good idea to avoid excessive salt in the diet but there is no evidence that going on a very low-salt diet helps. Do NOT take salt substitutes (high in potassium) without checking with your doctor, because

Daily intake of food types

Aim to balance your daily intake of the different food types into the approximate proportions shown above.

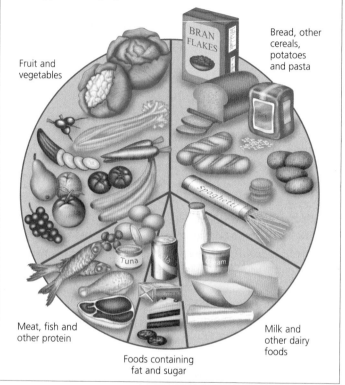

Fruit and vegetables

Bread, other cereals, potatoes and pasta

Meat, fish and other protein

Milk and other dairy foods

Foods containing fat and sugar

some treatments (angiotensin-converting enzyme or ACE inhibitors, angiotensin receptor blockers, spironolactone and eplerenone) can cause an excessive rise of potassium in the blood.

Some foods are obviously high in salt (crisps, salted nuts, pickles) but it is less obvious with many other foods (pizza, most curries, many tinned foods). Fresh and frozen foods generally have less salt.

Otherwise, you should try to have a 'healthy', well-balanced diet. You should avoid excessively fatty foods and ensure that you eat plenty of fruit and vegetables. If you feel that you could use some specific advice on how to improve your diet, ask to see a dietitian either at the health centre or at the hospital.

Alcohol

You may have been told that too much alcohol has caused damage to your heart muscle; in that case, total abstinence is the only sensible course. Otherwise, alcohol in moderation should do no harm, provided that you avoid 'binge' drinking.

Rest and exercise

Although you may need to rest in bed if your heart failure is severe or while your treatment is being stabilised, exercise is generally good for you. However, bed rest (lying down) helps kidney function. If you have severe heart failure, lying down for a few hours after taking your diuretic will make the medication work better. A daily regime, including a 'nap' in bed during the day for an hour or so and some regular exercise, such as a brisk walk, is probably ideal.

Whenever you can, make a point of getting some kind of exercise each day. Walking quickly, cycling and swimming are probably the best forms of exercise. You should exercise enough to make yourself mildly breathless but not do so much that it makes you feel ill.

When the weather is too bad or it's difficult to get out for some reason, making the beds or doing other housework at a smart pace is sufficiently demanding. If you have a local gym they may have exercise sessions for people with heart conditions. If you are worried about the safety of taking exercise your doctor may be able to organise a medically supervised exercise test.

There are some forms of exercise that you shouldn't try. In general, you should avoid lifting weights that are so heavy that they make you grunt or need you to hold your breath while lifting.

If you feel exhausted, develop chest pain or become very breathless you should stop and take a rest. Try to

Lifestyle changes

You can do a lot to help your long-term health by making simple lifestyle changes: maintain the correct weight for your height, stop smoking, drink alcohol in moderation, eat plenty of fruit and vegetables, and take regular exercise.

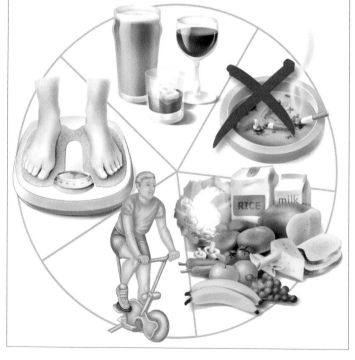

avoid situations that force you to do more exercise than you feel able to do. You should be able to choose when you want to stop. Don't try to run a marathon!

Taking your medication

Tablets work only if you take them. They do you no good in the bottle. However well intentioned you may be, it can be difficult to remember to take them so, if you have a problem, work out some way of reminding yourself or checking whether you have taken them.

For example, you could set your alarm clock (or even an alarm watch) for the appropriate time, or get hold of a proper pill dispenser from a pharmacy. Alternatively, make a simple pill dispenser for yourself from an egg box – just set out your day's dose each morning, then you can check later whether you've taken them. Make sure you keep them out of reach of children.

Remember that you may need to re-time your water tablets if you're going to be out and away from a toilet for some time. You should also leave enough time between taking your water pills and going to bed so that you do not have to get up too often at night. Other tablets should be taken at around the same time each day to keep the level of the medicine in your blood as constant as possible.

Should you notice any side effects from any of the medicines that you are taking, discuss the matter with your doctor. There are alternatives available in most cases, and sometimes it needs a bit of trial and error to find which ones suit you best. Make sure you organise a new supply before the old one runs out and that you always have enough to cover you for holidays.

Checking your progress

When you start treatment, you should notice an improvement in your symptoms. Breathlessness, in particular, should become less of a problem. You should also find you can gradually do a bit more as far as exercise is concerned as your stamina starts to come back. Water tablets usually improve symptoms quickly. ACE inhibitors may take weeks and beta blockers months to have their full effects. You may feel temporarily worse for a week or so after starting a beta blocker.

How you get on doing the same task is a useful gauge of how well your heart is working. Aim to set yourself at least one task to do three or four times a week – something that gets you mildly out of breath, like walking uphill to the shops. Don't overdo it so that you end up completely puffed. If at any time you notice yourself getting more out of breath doing the same walk, or that you seem to be able to do less and less, report this to your doctor.

Don't forget, however, that other illnesses could also be playing a part: for example, a chest infection will make you breathless and you'll feel tired after you've had the 'flu'.

Watch your weight

When heart failure is going out of control, relatively rapid weight change can occur and it's important that it's picked up as soon as possible. The point of weighing yourself each day is to check whether you are retaining too much fluid. You may recall from an earlier chapter that one litre of urine weighs one kilogram (that is, 2.2 pounds) so any sudden weight gain indicates that you may be retaining fluid.

What should you weigh?

- The body mass index (BMI) is a useful measure of healthy weight
- Find out your height in metres and weight in kilograms
- Calculate your BMI like this:

$$BMI = \frac{\text{Your weight (kg)}}{[\text{Your height (metres)} \times \text{Your height (metres)}]}$$

$$\text{e.g. } 24.8 = \frac{70}{[1.68 \times 1.68]}$$

- You are recommended to try to maintain a BMI in the range 18.5–24.9
- The chart below is an easier way of estimating your BMI. Read off your height and your weight. The point where the lines cross in the chart indicates your BMI

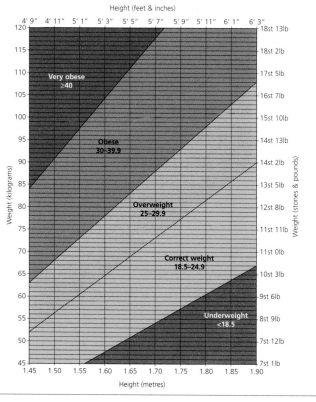

Tell your doctor if you gain more than two to three kilograms (four to six pounds) in a week. It sounds obvious, but you do need to be sure that you have a good, reliable set of bathroom scales and that they are standing on a hard and level surface (do NOT put the scales on a carpet!). You can't monitor your weight accurately otherwise.

Remember also that, if you're away from home and using different scales, the readings will almost certainly vary from the ones at home. The solution is to weigh yourself when you arrive at your destination, if possible, so you have a reference point against which to check any ups and downs in your weight.

The best time for your daily weigh-in is first thing, before getting dressed but after emptying your bladder. You should note your weight each day in a diary. Normally, you'll find that your weight varies very little from one day to the next, even if the long-term trend is up or down.

What makes heart failure worse?

There are a number of reasons why someone with heart failure may find that their condition is gradually getting worse:

- Forgetting to take medication
- Too much salt in the diet
- Taking medicines that can aggravate the problem, such as some treatments for arthritis and some painkillers
- The condition that originally caused your heart failure starts to get worse

- You develop some new problem with your heart, for example, if your heart rhythm becomes irregular, you may suddenly start feeling much worse and need new treatment

- Infections, usually in the chest or urine

- Anaemia, as a result of either iron deficiency or other causes (requires a blood test)

- Kidney problems (requires a blood test).

Inappropriate medicines
Taking some medicines can aggravate heart failure, for instance some treatments for arthritis and some painkillers. This includes some that you can buy without a prescription, such as ibuprofen, so always check with the pharmacist before buying anything that you haven't used before. The pharmacist will usually be able to suggest acceptable alternatives – paracetamol rather than ibuprofen, for example.

Some prescription medicines that you may have been taking for another heart condition – such as calcium channel blockers – may not be appropriate in people who have developed heart failure because they can make it worse. Do check with your doctor if you are unsure about any medicine you are taking.

Before starting any new course of medication make sure that you discuss with your doctor any existing medicines that you are taking – for possible adverse interactions. Carry a list of your medications (with doses) with you at all times in your wallet or purse.

Warning signs – and what to do
Chest pain
If you develop a crushing pain in your chest or down

your arms and into your jaw, rest in a sitting position. If you have GTN (glyceryl trinitrate) tablets to put under your tongue or a spray, ask someone to bring them to you if possible and use them immediately. If the pain hasn't gone after a few minutes, call an ambulance.

Palpitations

If you develop a fluttering feeling in your chest or feel your heart beating irregularly, rest for a while. If the feeling persists for more than 30 minutes or happens often, you should see your doctor. You may have occasional extra beats known as ectopics or intermittent atrial fibrillation (see page 24) and may need treatment.

Breathlessness

Sudden

If you wake up in the night severely short of breath, sit up and try to relax as much as you can. If the symptoms do not settle quickly, contact your doctor or, if he or she can't be reached within five minutes, phone the ambulance. You have probably got extra fluid on the lungs which needs to be treated promptly with an increased dose of diuretic medication, probably in the form of an injection. You may also need to be given oxygen.

Gradual

If you find your physical activity becoming increasingly limited and your breathlessness increasing, see your doctor. You may need to have your medication adjusted or to try a different treatment.

Weight gain

This may be a sign of increased fluid retention if it happens over a relatively short time, for example, two to three kilograms (four to six pounds) in a week or so (see page 61). See your doctor because you'll probably need to increase your dose of water tablets. If you can't see your doctor for some reason, take an extra water tablet each day until your weight returns to its usual level. However, you must report this to your doctor as soon as practical.

Weight loss

There are many reasons why people with heart failure lose weight, including development of diabetes or an overactive thyroid. It may also be a sign of worsening heart failure. If you are losing weight you should see your doctor.

Dizziness

This can be the result of low blood pressure, which may be a side effect of treatment, problems with the balance organs in the inner ear or heart rhythm problems. If you have persistent or severe dizziness or any form of blackout, you should see your doctor.

Dizziness that is caused by low blood pressure generally occurs when getting up from lying to standing position. You may be able to prevent it if you always remember to get up from lying down or sitting in stages – for example, when you're getting up in the morning, sit on the side of the bed for a minute before you stand up. This prevents your blood pressure from dropping suddenly. Should you have a dizzy spell or feel faint, lie down. It may help if you raise your legs a little by resting them on cushions or on a chair.

If this symptom is troublesome you should ask your practice nurse or doctor to check your blood pressure. Adjusting your medication (usually reducing the diuretic rather than the other treatments) may improve matters. For most patients who are not severely breathless a reduction in the dose of water tablets is worth a try. A bout of coughing or, in men, passing urine can trigger a drop in blood pressure and dizziness or even a blackout.

Dizziness caused by inner-ear problems is common and has many causes, most of which are not related directly to heart failure or its treatment. Causes include excessive ear wax, ear infection, a stroke or just stiffness that can develop in the organ of balance in the inner ear. This sort of dizziness is often made worse by a sudden movement of the head and can be made transiently worse by lying down (as well as standing up). It is often accompanied by nausea, especially if persistent. It does not cause blackouts. You should have your ears checked by a doctor. Regular exercises involving rotating and turning the head to loosen up the balance organ can help.

Heart rhythm problems usually cause dizziness to develop out of the blue and may be accompanied by palpitations and blackouts. These symptoms will usually last only a short time. Again you need to see your doctor.

KEY POINTS

- Don't smoke

- Eat a healthy diet (avoid excess salt)

- Take a sensible amount of exercise

- Drink alchohol only in moderation

- Take your medicines accurately

- Weigh yourself (and record your weight) regularly

- Keep a list of your medications (with doses) with you at all times in your purse or wallet

Living with heart failure

Understand your condition

Anyone who has a condition such as heart failure that cannot usually be completely cured will gradually learn from experience how he or she can best cope with it. As a general rule, the more you understand about what is wrong and why you get the symptoms that you do, the more you can help to minimise them, even if they can't be prevented altogether.

You need to know what has caused your heart failure and how it's being treated. You should know the purpose of any medication that you are taking, the right time of day to take it and what side effects, if any, to watch for. Make sure that you are clear about when and in what circumstances you need to call your doctor, other than for routine appointments.

It helps enormously if you can build up a good relationship with your GP and with any specialist who's treating you. It is important for you to feel that you can ask any questions that you want and contact the doctors for advice when you feel in need of it. You can help them to help you by not missing appointments unnecessarily and by keeping notes of any questions, minor changes in your condition or your response to treatment, so that you don't forget anything when you next see them.

Self-monitoring

Your doctors have to rely on you to let them know how you are doing on a day-to-day basis – which is why it's important to get into the habit of monitoring your condition. This means regular daily weigh-ins as outlined on page 94, as well as noting any changes in how much you can do or in other symptoms.

Take regular exercise

You will feel the benefit of regular daily exercise – enough to leave you feeling mildly breathless, but not too much – so doing something like a brisk walk every day is ideal. Try to manage some exercise at least three times a week.

Reduce stress

Depending on how you lived before you developed heart failure, you may need to give some thought to the amount of stress in your life and how you deal with it. Few of us can avoid stressful situations entirely, but it may be possible to reduce stress in your life to some extent. Many local education authorities run day-time or evening classes in relaxation or stress management and you can also buy cassettes designed to promote relaxation. For some people, work is stressful but, for others, retirement is even more so. Whether to give up work is a personal decision.

Self-monitoring

Get into the habit of monitoring your condition. Weigh yourself and note any changes in how you feel or how much you can do on a daily basis. Photocopy or make and complete a weekly chart.

Date	Day	Weight (early morning, empty bladder)

Medicine name	Dose	Frequency

Self-monitoring

Get into the habit of monitoring your condition. Weigh yourself and note any changes in how you feel or how much you can do on a daily basis. Photocopy or make and complete a weekly chart.

Week no. [   ]

How I feel (at the end of the day)

Other comments

Stop smoking

It cannot be said too often that smoking can only add to your problems if you have heart failure. Do ask your doctor for practical advice as well as the addresses and telephone numbers of organisations that can give you information and support when you want to stop smoking.

Eat sensibly

Your doctor should also be able to fill any gaps in your knowledge about the right kind of diet or arrange for you to have a chat with a dietitian if necessary. Eating properly can give a boost to your overall health, even if you don't need to worry about losing weight. And if you could do with shedding some excess fat, it's sensible to get a dietitian's advice on how to lose it slowly without going hungry or missing out on essential nutrients. Remember that carrying too much extra weight puts added strain on your heart, and makes any kind of exercise more difficult.

Alcohol

Having heart failure doesn't mean that you have to give up all your former pleasures! Unless your heart failure was actually the result of damage caused by excessive drinking, you don't have to give up alcohol. Moderate drinking won't do any harm, although beer drinkers may need to watch the volume of liquid they consume if they are prone to fluid retention.

Sex

Some people are also concerned that their heart problem may curtail their sex life. In fact, the only aspect of heart failure that might affect your ability to make love is being short of breath. Otherwise, there is no reason why you shouldn't have sex whenever you and your partner feel like it. The only exception is during the period immediately after a heart attack, when you should abstain from sex for about six weeks to allow the heart to heal. For men who have difficulty getting an erection, Viagra (sildenafil) appears safe provided that it is not given with nitrates. Seek medical advice.

Travel and holidays

If you're planning a long journey or stay away from home, it's a good idea to have a word with your doctor beforehand. Anyone travelling outside the UK needs good travel insurance. You may find that many of the standard policies don't cover you for conditions that you already know about when you take them out – such as heart failure. Should you encounter difficulties with insurance, contact the British Heart Foundation (address on page 121) which can give you a list of insurance companies sympathetic to those with heart complaints. Before you leave home, you should also check with your GP whether you need any immunisations or to take tablets to protect you against malaria, for example.

Unless your heart failure is severe, your doctor will probably encourage you in your plans. You will need to take particular care if your destination is very hot or very cold, and people with more than mild heart failure are normally advised not to visit high-altitude resorts – those over 2,000 metres (6,000 feet) – because there is less oxygen in the atmosphere. You needn't be put off by the prospect of long flights provided that you plan ahead and follow some commonsense rules while you're away.

How to travel

Having decided on your destination, you may or may not have any real choice about what means of transport you use to get there. When you do have options, however, or the journey is a factor in choosing where to go, you need to work out your priorities. For example, a car is the ideal choice if your main concern is to be able to travel at your own pace and stop whenever you want. On the other hand, long journeys by car can be stressful, especially if you're the only driver. Trains and even coaches have toilets on board and you can get up and stretch your legs if you want. Travelling by sea is relaxing – provided that you're not prone to sea-sickness! If you are, it's worth taking antihistamine patches with you or wearing them all the time you're on board if necessary.

It is best to try out sea-sickness medication in advance to make sure that it gives you no side effects (such as palpitations, dizziness, dry mouth, blurred vision). Remember that sickness can lead to a reduction in your salt and fluid levels and prevent you absorbing medication, so it's important to avoid it if you can.

Flying may be the most convenient as well as the fastest way to your destination, but airports can be very stressful as well as involving long treks to the departure gates. The level of oxygen in aircraft cabins is lower than normal, but this is not usually a problem unless heart failure is severe.

On long flights, you must take care not to become dehydrated, especially if you are taking diuretic tablets or ACE inhibitors. You should steer clear of alcohol because it increases the risk of dehydration and try to move around the aircraft at least once every hour or so if you can, to stop blood clots forming in the legs. Most

Holiday checkpoints

- Talk to your doctor before you go and discuss how to tackle potential problems. In particular, make sure you understand what to do if your weight increases or drops suddenly while you're away.

- Make sure you have adequate health insurance cover and that it does not exclude 'pre-existing' conditions such as heart failure.

- Check that scales will be available at your destination and, if not, consider making room for a set in your luggage.

- If you're travelling by sea or air, let the airline or shipping company know that you have heart failure when you book.

- Keep a close eye on your weight while you're away and be prepared to adjust your medication, salt and fluid intake in case of any sudden changes.

- Take sensible precautions to protect your health – don't overdo the alcohol and steer clear of any food or drink liable to provoke tummy upsets. In countries where hygiene standards may be dubious, avoid ice cream, shellfish, fruit that needs washing rather than peeling, and salads and ice (unless from bottled water).

- Always protect your skin against the sun and, if taking amiodarone, apply a total block before going out in the sun.

airline magazines recommend a series of leg stretching exercises. You are strongly advised to comply with these.

It's a wise precaution to let the airline know that you have a heart failure, if it is severe, when you book so that they can make supplementary oxygen available just in case. You can also book a wheelchair if you need it, and most UK airports now offer a buggy service to get you to the plane if necessary, but you need to check whether this is also available at your destination airport.

When you arrive
Monitor your weight
As soon as you arrive you should weigh yourself. Either check in advance with the hotel that they have scales or pack you own (provided that there is someone else to carry your bag!). You may well find that the result is different from your home scales, so use this as your reference point – all scales vary. You may be eating quite a different diet from usual, so you need to keep an eye on your salt and fluid balance. Continue to weigh yourself daily and, if your weight drops by more than three kilograms, you'll need to take action. It means that you are short of fluid, so if you're on water tablets stop taking them for the time being. Otherwise, eat salty foods – such as salted nuts and crisps – and drink non-alcoholic fluids until your weight comes back up to within two to three kilograms of your target weight before restarting your water pills. Try not to over-compensate. You should avoid excessive weight gain.

Stomach and bowel upsets
Remember that if you have a tummy upset with diarrhoea and/or vomiting, you can easily become dehydrated. If severe, you need to stop taking water tablets and ACE inhibitors for a while, and drink lots of non-alcoholic drinks. Keep weighing yourself until the scales tell you that your fluid balance is nearly back to normal, when you can restart your usual medicines.

Don't hesitate to see a local doctor if you don't feel able to handle the situation on your own. Remember that vomiting, diarrhoea and sweating can also lead to salt depletion, which may lead to muscle cramps.

Sunburn

Sunburn – and even a suntan – is a sign that your skin is being damaged by exposure to the sun and excessive exposure should be avoided. Amiodarone can increase the sensitivity to sunlight and, because this increase in sensitivity is not confined to ultraviolet light, normal suncreams do not work.

People with very fair skin, especially red-head, Celtic types, are especially likely to have this problem. The longer amiodarone is taken, the more likely it is to occur. If you are taking amiodarone, the first question to ask is whether you still need to take it. Discuss this with your doctor.

Even if you can stop amiodarone, it will take a year or more before this problem goes away if you have been taking the treatment for a long time, because it is stored in the body for a long time. Avoiding strong sunlight by staying indoors or wearing a sunhat and long sleeves or using a total sun-block (ask your pharmacist) will help you avoid this problem.

Your family and friends

Family and friends can't help being concerned about your condition, but they may worry less if they can learn more about it. Obviously, individuals vary as to how much detail they want to know. The last thing you need from those close to you is gloom and doom, and they will find it far easier to adopt a positive approach when they know something about your condition and treatment. You will probably rely on their moral support on days when you are feeling less well so the more they understand the better. Most people want the answers to a few basic questions.

What is heart failure?

The term sounds rather dramatic and some people think that it means your heart is going to stop at any moment. This is not the case. It will probably help to read the introductory section on pages 1–7.

How does it affect you?

People you spend a lot of time with or see regularly need to know about any limitations that your condition places on you. For example, the fact that you can't perhaps walk as far or as fast as you once did or can no longer do heavy gardening or carry heavy shopping.

Will it get worse?

Most people with heart failure find it easier to cope if they have someone they can rely on if they get new symptoms or old ones return. Explain to them what symptoms could affect you, such as increased breathlessness or problems with your fluid balance, and what needs doing in a given set of circumstances, for example, reduce the amount of salt in the diet if weight is increasing or perhaps increase the dose of diuretic (but please tell your doctor or nurse if you have had to do this on more than a few occasions). It can also be a big help if someone else remembers to check that you have taken your medicines correctly!

What should a relative or friend do in an emergency?

It may never happen, but someone who has been on a first aid course that includes basic resuscitation techniques will feel much more confident about coping in a crisis. A basic 'save-a-life' course takes only two hours. If they know what to do when someone loses consciousness while waiting for the ambulance, they could save someone's life one day! Contact the St John Ambulance (see page 125).

Who is at risk?

Knowing that you have heart failure may lead your relatives to worry whether they may develop the same problem one day. Anyone who is worried should explain the situation to his or her doctor, giving as much information about your condition as possible. The GP will then be able to advise him or her as to whether any investigations are necessary.

It may be necessary for close family members to have regular blood pressure or cholesterol checks, and they may be told that smoking presents even greater risks for them than for others. In some cases, relatives will need to have an ECG or echocardiogram (see pages 46 and 47). However, it's quite likely that they will be told that their risk of developing heart failure is not increased just because you have it.

Looking to the future

The outlook for someone with heart failure will vary depending on what has caused it. For example, when it is the result of atrial fibrillation or valve disease, the underlying problem can often be cured so that the

Basic resuscitation – the recovery position for an unconscious adult

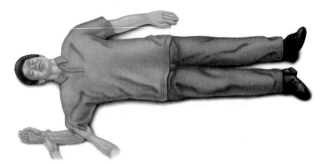

1. (a) Kneel beside the casualty.
   (b) Remove spectacles and any bulky items from pockets.
   (c) Straighten legs.
   (d) Place the arm nearest to you at right angles to the body.

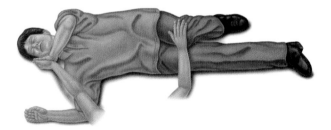

2. (a) Bring the arm furthest from you across the casualty's chest and hold the back of his hand against the cheek nearest to you.
   (b) Using your other hand, grasp the furthest leg just above the knee and raise it up until the foot is flat on the floor.

Basic resuscitation – the recovery position for an unconscious adult (contd)

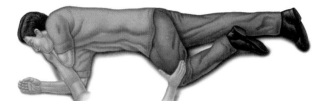

3. Keeping the casualty's hand pressed against his cheek, pull on the far leg and roll him towards you and on to his side.

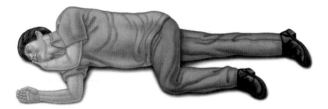

4. (a) Adjust the upper leg so that both the knee and hip are bent at right angles.

 (b) Tilt the head back to ensure the airway remains open.

 (c) Ensure the hand remains under the cheek, helping to keep the airway open.

ABC of resuscitation

The ABC stands for 'Airway', 'Breathing' and 'Circulation'. The following procedure is only an outline of the techniques that may be of use to assist an unconscious adult before emergency help arrives.

If you wish to be well prepared for an emergency, undertake an accredited first aid course.

Airway
Place one hand on the casualty's forehead. Tilt the head back and the mouth will fall open.

Remove any obvious obstructions from the mouth.

To open the airway, lift the chin with the fingertips of your other hand. Is the casualty now breathing?

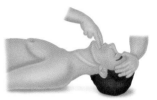

Breathing
Watch the chest for movement, listen for sounds of breathing and feel for breath on your cheek.

If breathing is absent give two rescue breaths (see later), then check for signs of circulation and call for emergency help.

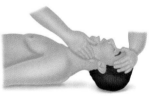

Circulation
You will have called for emergency help by this stage.

Check the pulse in the neck for 5–10 seconds – see diagram.

If signs of circulation are absent start chest compression (CPR) with rescue breaths.

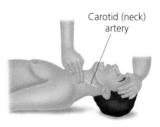

Carotid (neck) artery

Cardiopulmonary resuscitation (CPR)

CPR is a life-saving technique in which artificial respiration is combined with chest compression to force oxygenated blood around the body. Undertake an accredited course if you wish to master the technique.

Chest compressions

Modern guidelines emphasise the importance of chest compressions for resuscitation of someone who has no pulse or heart beat and is not breathing. The number and duration of pauses should be kept to a minimum.

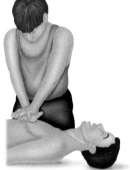

Make a diagnosis of cardiac arrest if a victim is unresponsive, has no detectable pulse and is not breathing normally. Patients whose hearts have stopped may still make occasional gasping breaths.

Place your hands in the centre of the chest over the breast bone (sternum).

Give 30 chest compressions immediately then try to give 2 short rescue breaths lasting 1–2 seconds each. If you feel unable to give rescue breaths then just continue with compressions. Compressions of adequate rate and depth (2–4 cm or about 3 inches) with full-chest recoil and minimal interruptions are required. For periods of up to 5 minutes compressions alone can save a life.

Ideally, use a ratio of 30 compressions to 2 rescue breaths (ventilations). There should be no longer than 10 seconds between one set of compressions and the next.

Rescue breaths

Pinch the soft part of the nose to seal it. Open the casualty's mouth.

Take a deep breath that fills your lungs.

Place your open mouth tightly around the casualty's open mouth to create a good seal. Place a handkerchief over the victim's mouth if this helps you.

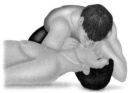

Blow air steadily into the casualty's mouth for about 2 seconds – the chest should rise.

Remove your mouth and the casualty's chest should fall.

individual's prospects are similar to those of anyone else of around the same age.

When the cause cannot be corrected in this way, the outlook may be less favourable. This is the case for most people whose heart failure is caused by a heart attack, high blood pressure or heart muscle disease.

Twenty years ago most people could expect to survive with heart failure for only a few years. Thanks to recent advances in medical care, many people with heart failure are surviving much, much longer, provided that they get expert investigations and advice and follow the latter.

Modern combination treatment has increased life expectancy with heart failure by two to three times. Treatment is much more effective if started early. New and effective treatments mean that even some people with heart muscle disease can be cured (although they may still require life-long treatment to prevent recurrence).

Treatment not only prolongs life but also usually improves the quality of life. Although you may get side effects from treatment, in the long run most patients feel worse if they do not take their medication.

KEY POINTS

■ It is fine to travel abroad as long as you take sensible precautions

■ Make sure you know how to deal with dehydration (diarrhoea and vomiting)

■ It is good to travel with a friend/relative who understands your condition in case of emergency

Useful addresses

We have included the following organisations because, on preliminary investigation, they may be of use to the reader. However, we do not have first-hand experience of each organisation and so cannot guarantee the organisation's integrity. The reader must therefore exercise his or her own discretion and judgement when making further enquiries.

Benefits Enquiry Line
Tel: 0800 882200
Minicom: 0800 243355
Website: www.dwp.gov.uk
N. Ireland: 0800 220674

Government agency giving information and advice on sickness and disability benefits for people with disabilities and their carers.

Blood Pressure Association
60 Cranmer Terrace
London SW17 0QS
Tel: 020 8772 4994

Information helpline: 0845 241 0989 (11am–3pm,
Mon–Fri)
Website: www.bpassoc.org.uk

Raises public awareness about, and offers information
and support to, people affected by high blood pressure
and health-care professionals. Has a wide selection of
literature and free membership scheme.

British Heart Foundation
14 Fitzhardinge Street
London W1H 6DH
Tel: 020 7935 0185
Helpline: 08450 708070 (Mon, Tues, Fri 9am–5pm,
Wed, Thurs 8am–6pm)
Website: www.bhf.org.uk
Publications' order line: 0870 600 6566

Funds research, promotes education and raises money
to buy equipment to treat heart disease. Information
and support available for people with heart conditions.
Via Heartstart UK arranges training in emergency life-
saving techniques for lay people.

Cardiomyopathy Association
Unit 10, Chiltern Court, Asheridge Road
Chesham, Bucks HP5 2PX
Tel: 01494 791224
Helpline: 0800 018 1024
Website: www.cardiomyopathy.org

Support organisation helping patients and medical
professionals with information on hypertrophic, dilated
and other forms of cardiomyopathy.

Clinical Knowledge Summaries

Sowerby Centre for Health Informatics at Newcastle
(SCHIN Ltd), Bede House, All Saints Business Centre
Newcastle upon Tyne NE1 2ES
Tel: 0191 243 6100
Website: www.cks.library.nhs.uk

A website mainly for GPs giving information for patients
listed by disease plus named self-help organisations.

Diabetes UK

Macleod House, 10 Parkway
London NW1 7AA
Tel: 020 7424 1000
Helpline: 0845 120 2960 (Mon–Fri, 9am–5pm)
Website: www.diabetes.org.uk

Provides advice and information for people with
diabetes and their families. Has local support groups.

Disabled Living Foundation

380–384 Harrow Road
London W9 2HU
Tel: 020 7289 6111
Helpline: 0845 130 9177
Textphone 020 7432 8009
Website: www.dlf.org.uk

Provides information to disabled and elderly people on
all kinds of equipment in order to promote their
independence and quality of life.

DVLA

Driver and Vehicle Licensing Agency

Swansea SA6 7JL
Tel: 0870 600 0301
Website: www.dvla.gov.uk

Contact the DVLA if you suffer from heart failure.
Provides information about medical conditions, driving
licences, learning to drive, entitlement to drive,
endorsements/disqualifications, driving abroad and what
to do when you have changed your address and/or name.

HEART UK
7 North Road
Maidenhead, Berks SL6 1PE
Tel: 0845 450 5988
Website: www.heartuk.org.uk

Offers information, advice and support to people with
coronary heart disease and especially those at high risk
of familial hypercholesterolaemia. Members receive
bimonthly magazine.

Lifesavers, The Royal Life Saving Society UK
River House, High Street
Broom, Warwickshire B50 4HN
Tel: 01789 773994
Website: www.lifesavers.org.uk

Runs courses throughout the UK in water safety,
rescue techniques and life support.

National Institute for Health and Clinical Excellence (NICE)
MidCity Place, 71 High Holborn
London WC1V 6NA

Tel: 0845 003 7780
Website: www.nice.org.uk

Provides national guidance on the promotion of good health and the prevention and treatment of ill-health. Patient information leaflets are available for each piece of guidance issued.

NHS Direct
Tel: 0845 4647 (24 hours, 365 days a year)
Website: www.nhsdirect.nhs.uk

Offers confidential health-care advice, information and referral service. A good first port of call for any health advice.

NHS Smoking Helpline
Freephone: 0800 169 0169 (7am–11pm, 365 days a year)
Website: www.givingupsmoking.co.uk
Pregnancy smoking helpline: 0800 169 9169 (7am–11pm, 365 days a year)

Have advice, help and encouragement on giving up smoking. Specialist advisers available to offer ongoing support to those who genuinely are trying to give up smoking. Can refer to local branches.

Patients' Association
PO Box 935
Harrow, Middlesex HA1 3YJ
Helpline: 0845 608 4455
Tel: 020 8423 9111
Website: www.patients-association.com

Provides advice on patients' rights, leaflets and a directory of self-help groups.

Quit (Smoking Quitlines)
211 Old Street
London EC1V 9NR
Tel: 020 7251 1551
Helpline: 0800 002200 (9am–9pm, 365 days a year)
Website: www.quit.org.uk
Scotland: 0800 848484
Wales: 0800 169 0169 (NHS)

Offers individual advice on giving up smoking in English and Asian languages. Talks to schools on smoking and pregnancy and can refer to local support groups. Runs training courses for professionals.

Resuscitation Council (UK)
5th Floor, Tavistock House North, Tavistock Square
London WC1H 9HR
Tel: 020 7388 4678
Website: www.resus.org.uk

Sets standards and runs courses for health-care professionals. Sells publications on resuscitation and funds research.

St John Ambulance
27 St John's Lane
London EC1M 4BU
Tel: 020 7324 4000
Helpline: 08700 104950 (office hours)
Website: www.sja.org.uk

Provides training locally throughout the UK and first aid at public events via its members. Offers a variety of welfare services in local communities.

Useful websites
BBC
www.bbc.co.uk/health
A helpful website: easy to navigate and offers lots of useful advice and information. Also contains links to other related topics.

Patient UK
www.patient.co.uk
Patient care website.

The internet as a source of further information
After reading this book, you may feel that you would like further information on the subject. The internet is of course an excellent place to look and there are many websites with useful information about medical disorders, related charities and support groups.

It should always be remembered, however, that the internet is unregulated and anyone is free to set up a website and add information to it. Many websites offer impartial advice and information that have been compiled and checked by qualified medical professionals. Some, on the other hand, are run by commercial organisations with the purpose of promoting their own products. Others still are run by pressure groups, some of which will provide carefully assessed and accurate information whereas others may be suggesting medications or treatments that are not supported by the medical and scientific community.

Unless you know the address of the website you want to visit – for example, www.familydoctor.co.uk – you may find the following guidelines useful when searching the internet for information.

Search engines and other searchable sites

Google (www.google.co.uk) is the most popular search engine used in the UK, followed by Yahoo! (http://uk.yahoo.com) and MSN (www.msn.co.uk). Also popular are the search engines provided by Internet Service Providers such as Tiscali and other sites such as the BBC site (www.bbc.co.uk).

In addition to the search engines that index the whole web, there are also medical sites with search facilities, which act almost like mini-search engines, but cover only medical topics or even a particular area of medicine. Again, it is wise to look at who is responsible for compiling the information offered to ensure that it is impartial and medically accurate. The NHS Direct site (www.nhsdirect.nhs.uk) is an example of a searchable medical site.

Links to many British medical charities can be found at the Association of Medical Research Charities' website (www. amrc.org.uk) and at Charity Choice (www. charitychoice.co.uk).

Search phrases

Be specific when entering a search phrase. Searching for information on 'cancer' will return results for many different types of cancer as well as on cancer in general. You may even find sites offering astrological information. More useful results will be returned by using search phrases such as 'lung cancer' and 'treatments for lung cancer'. Both Google and Yahoo!

offer an advanced search option that includes the ability to search for the exact phrase; enclosing the search phrase in quotes, that is, 'treatments for lung cancer', will have the same effect. Limiting a search to an exact phrase reduces the number of results returned but it is best to refine a search to an exact match only if you are not getting useful results with a normal search. Adding 'UK' to your search term will bring up mainly British sites, so a good phrase might be 'lung cancer' UK (don't include UK within the quotes).

Always remember the internet is international and unregulated. It holds a wealth of valuable information but individual sites may be biased, out of date or just plain wrong. Family Doctor Publications accepts no responsibility for the content of links published in this series.

Index

Your pages

We have included the following pages because they may help you manage your illness or condition and its treatment.

Before an appointment with a health professional, it can be useful to write down a short list of questions of things that you do not understand, so that you can make sure that you do not forget anything.

Some of the sections may not be relevant to your circumstances.

We are always pleased to receive constructive criticism or suggestions about how to improve the books. You can contact us at:

Email: familydoctor@btinternet.com
Letter: Family Doctor Publications
        PO Box 4664
        Poole
        BH15 1NN

Thank you

Health-care contact details

Name:

Job title:

Place of work:

Tel:

Name:

Job title:

Place of work:

Tel:

Name:

Job title:

Place of work:

Tel:

Name:

Job title:

Place of work:

Tel:

Significant past health events – illnesses/ operations/investigations/treatments

Event	Month	Year	Age (at time)

Appointments for health care

Name:

Place:

Date:

Time:

Tel:

Name:

Place:

Date:

Time:

Tel:

Name:

Place:

Date:

Time:

Tel:

Name:

Place:

Date:

Time:

Tel:

Appointments for health care

Name:

Place:

Date:

Time:

Tel:

Name:

Place:

Date:

Time:

Tel:

Name:

Place:

Date:

Time:

Tel:

Name:

Place:

Date:

Time:

Tel:

Current medication(s) prescribed by your doctor

Medicine name:

Purpose:

Frequency & dose:

Start date:

End date:

Medicine name:

Purpose:

Frequency & dose:

Start date:

End date:

Medicine name:

Purpose:

Frequency & dose:

Start date:

End date:

Medicine name:

Purpose:

Frequency & dose:

Start date:

End date:

Other medicines/supplements you are taking, not prescribed by your doctor

Medicine/treatment:

Purpose:

Frequency & dose:

Start date:

End date:

Medicine/treatment:

Purpose:

Frequency & dose:

Start date:

End date:

Medicine/treatment:

Purpose:

Frequency & dose:

Start date:

End date:

Medicine/treatment:

Purpose:

Frequency & dose:

Start date:

End date:

Questions to ask at appointments
(Note: do bear in mind that doctors work under great time pressure, so long lists may not be helpful for either of you)

Questions to ask at appointments
(Note: do bear in mind that doctors work under great time pressure, so long lists may not be helpful for either of you)

Notes